RAND NATIONAL DEFENSE RESEARCH INSTITUTE

Suicide Postvention in the Department of Defense

Evidence, Policies and Procedures, and Perspectives of Loss Survivors

Rajeev Ramchand, Lynsay Ayer, Gail Fisher, Karen Chan Osilla,
Dionne Barnes-Proby, Samuel Wertheimer

Prepared for the Office of the Secretary of Defense

For more information on this publication, visit www.rand.org/t/RR586

Library of Congress Cataloging-in-Publication Data is available for this publication.
ISBN: 978-0-8330-8642-6

Published by the RAND Corporation, Santa Monica, Calif.

Cover: U.S Air Force photo by Airman 1st Class Shannon Hall

Preface

The suicide rate in the U.S. armed forces has almost doubled over the past decade. In response, a number of studies and initiatives have focused on preventing suicide among service members. Consistent across this research is the notion that while preventing suicide is paramount, responding to military suicides is equally important.

To help the U.S. Department of Defense (DoD) craft policies and procedures to better respond to suicides in its ranks, the Defense Centers of Excellence for Psychological Health and Traumatic Brain Injury asked the RAND National Defense Research Institute to do the following:

- Collect pertinent information on policies and procedures in DoD and across the military services for responding to service member deaths generally and suicide specifically.
- Document the extent to which DoD programs and policies reflect state-of-the-art suicide postvention practices.
- Provide a snapshot of how installations across the services respond to suicides.
- Develop recommendations for DoD to improve its response to suicides.

This report presents the result of that effort. It was prepared specifically for military leaders, chaplains, behavioral health professionals, and other key personnel who are often involved in responding to a suicide. However, the results may be of interest to both federal and nongovernmental organizations that are also called upon to provide services or otherwise respond to the tragic event of a service member taking his or her life. Importantly, this report attempts to systematically describe what organizations can hope to achieve by crafting a coordinated response to a suicide, what recommendations have been put forth to help organizations craft such a response, and what science exists to support those recommendations.

This research was sponsored by the Defense Centers of Excellence for Psychological Health and Traumatic Brain Injury and conducted within the Forces and Resources Policy Center of the RAND National Defense Research Institute, a federally funded research and development center sponsored by the Office of the Secretary of Defense, the Joint Staff, the Unified Combatant Commands, the Navy, the Marine Corps, the defense agencies, and the defense Intelligence Community.

For more information on the Forces and Resources Policy Center, see http://www.rand.org/nsrd/ndri/centers/frp.html or contact the director (contact information is provided on the web page).

Contents

Figure and Tables

Figures

Tables

Summary

Background and Purpose

The U.S. Department of Defense (DoD) has always been concerned about suicides among service members, and the increase in suicides over the past decade has heightened that concern. Previously, DoD asked the RAND Center for Military Health Policy Research to identify best suicide prevention practices and ascertain whether the military services' suicide prevention programs used them. The results of that research were reported in *The War Within: Preventing Suicide in the U.S. Military* (Ramchand, Acosta, et al., 2011), which recommended that DoD provide formal guidance to commanders about how to respond to suicides among military personnel. This report aims to help DoD create such guidance, and it does so in three ways.

First, this report critically reviews the scientific evidence to date on how to respond to suicide across four domains: surveillance, preventing subsequent suicides, grief support, and respecting and honoring the deceased and his or her loved ones. It then presents current DoD policies and practices in each domain to identify gaps and opportunities for improvement.

Second, in compiling this report it became apparent that there is little scientific evidence on how best to respond to suicides. However, there is a series of resource guides to which DoD leaders may turn. We reviewed a large number of these resource guides and describe systematically what they recommend and what research evidence exists to support these recommendations.

Third, we wanted to assess how DoD and installations respond to suicide in practice. To do so, we conducted a qualitative study to learn more about the experiences of military suicide loss survivors through focus groups at a national loss survivor conference.[1]

We chose this multimethod approach to provide a comprehensive review of postvention policies and procedures informed by a variety of perspectives. For example, the scientific literature may help identify which postvention programs have been shown to be effective. However, a review of DoD policies and procedures is necessary to determine whether and how such programs are or could be implemented in the military. Our review of the resource guides also helped identify other promising approaches in need of scientific testing. Focus groups with friends and family members of personnel who have died by suicide helped us understand the impact, costs, and benefits of current DoD postvention policies and procedures. We incorporated all these perspectives into 12 recommendations that DoD or its suborganizations could adopt to strengthen their responses to suicide.

[1] Throughout this report, we use the phrase *loss survivors* to refer to the family and friends of a person who has taken his or her own life.

How DoD Policies and Procedures Map onto the Research Evidence and Resource Guidelines and Recommendations

Surveillance

Suicide surveillance is defined as the tracking and reporting of information related to suicide, and accurate surveillance enables policymakers and practitioners to respond to trends or design targeted interventions. Suicide surveillance is challenging due to variability in the degree to which suspected suicides are investigated, jurisdictional variation in the requirements for making a suicide determination, and regional differences in how equivocal deaths—or those for which the cause of death is indeterminate—are investigated. Primarily based on expert opinions, the evidence provides guidance to medical examiners in making cause-of-death determinations, determining which core data elements should be included in surveillance systems, and deciding how to conduct psychological autopsy studies. Resource guides offer few recommendations regarding surveillance; those that do generally stress the importance of preparing to respond to a suicide before one occurs and incorporating surveillance activities in such a plan, or the importance of treating loss survivors with sensitivity during death-scene investigations.

Data on military suicides derive from military criminal investigations, autopsies conducted by the Armed Forces Medical Examiner System, and command-directed investigations (i.e., line-of-duty [LoD] investigations). The purpose of LoD investigations is to ascertain whether an event occurred due to negligence or misconduct on the part of the service member. Suicide deaths among active-duty personnel are generally determined to occur "in the line of duty," though they may be considered "not in the line of duty" if the investigating officer presents evidence of mental soundness on the part of the service member who died. Such determination affects loss survivors' eligibility for benefits provided by both DoD and the U.S. Department of Veterans Affairs (VA).

DoD's suicide surveillance activities are centered on the recently established DoD Suicide Event Report (DoDSER). These surveillance efforts are standardized for service members on active duty, but suicides in the National Guard and reserves are not tracked in a consistent way and often rely on civilian cause-of-death determinations and surveillance. DoDSER surveillance efforts generally surpass those in civilian settings, particularly for active-duty suicides. The DoDSER data elements have heavy overlap with the core elements recommended by national guidelines. However, noticeably absent is a field identifying the source of each DoDSER data element. Given the different sources from which data may derive, combining data elements from multiple sources and treating all data fields as equally valid and reliable could create biases in how similar constructs are reported and analyzed.

Suicide Prevention After a Suicide Death

There is evidence that surviving family, friends, and colleagues may be at increased risk for suicide after a suicide death. There is also evidence of associations between media coverage of celebrity suicides and suicide rates among the general population. With respect to media coverage, associations are strongest for "authentic" coverage versus fictional portrayals in magazines or television shows, accounts in daily newspapers, and sensationalistic coverage.

No randomized controlled trials of interventions implemented immediately after a suicide have shown reductions in suicide deaths or interruptions of suicide clusters. However, panels of experts have established guidelines for how communities should respond to suicides and for how media should report on suicides. In the case of community responses, there is one published study showing that community adoption of an intervention was associated with a subsequent reduction in suicides (Hacker et al., 2003). Other postvention models exist and include an approach focused on consoling loss survivors at the death scene (which may lead to increased referral to supportive resources) and training community members to act as gatekeepers following a suicide. There is less evidence that adhering to certain media guidelines is effective.

Evidence from suicide prevention strategies more generally may be relevant and could be applied to help guide postvention activities. Universal screening for suicide risk in school settings has been able to identify persons who are thinking about suicide but who have not asked for help on their own or who have not been identified by school personnel. Such approaches may be relevant to DoD. In addition, the delivery of high-quality behavioral health care has been associated with reductions in suicides and nonfatal attempts. It is not known whether DoD is providing evidence-based care consistent with research recommendations for preventing suicide among those receiving treatment.

Resource guide recommendations related to preventing suicides after a suicide focus largely on having a plan for discussing suicide in advance, a process for identifying individuals at potentially increased risk, and communication guidelines that generally adhere to the recommendations for media coverage of suicide. In addition, there are recommendations to enhance or rejuvenate suicide prevention programs.

DoD currently has no policies or procedures addressing what to do after a suicide death to prevent subsequent suicides, and there is a limited evidence base to describe the state of the art in this area. Thus, it is virtually impossible to assess how DoD practices map onto state-of-the-art postvention procedures to prevent suicide. However, DoD, the services, and military organizations have responded to aggregate and noticeable increases in suicide rates or numbers in three ways. First, they have revised their existing suicide prevention programs. For example, the Air Force Suicide Prevention Program was created after a period of increasing suicides in the Air Force and reinvigorated after a later increase. Second, they have held mandatory "stand-downs," requiring large groups (or an entire service) to focus all or part of a day on suicide prevention or resilience-building. Third, they have evaluated their existing approaches to suicide prevention.

Grief Support After a Suicide

It is expected that loss survivors will experience a profound sense of loss and grief after a suicide. Although there is no evidence to date that those who experience a suicide loss display a unique form of grief, for some, the grief may become debilitating and reach the threshold of what is termed "complicated grief." There is no evidence to date on how complicated grief can be prevented, but there are evidence-based methods for treating complicated grief, primarily through cognitive behavioral therapy.

We found that resource guidelines regarding grief support fell in two general areas. First, there were recommendations for counselors and other support personnel to stress that loss survivors grieve differently and to expect differences in how loss survivors process their loved one's death. In addition, there were recommendations about caring for care providers, as counseling bereaved individuals can lead to compassion fatigue and distress. There were also communication guidelines, including how organizations should reach out to loss survivors, though there is no evidence to suggest that one method is better than another. Recommendations regarding memorial services often conflicted with each other; again, there is no evidence to suggest whether organizations should have memorial services or what these services should entail.

Other recommendations were similar to those for suicide prevention, including having plans prepared in advance and a process for identifying bereaved individuals at high risk for mental health problems and suicide.

DoD offers various resources to help loss survivors grieve. Casualty assistance officers (CAOs) are resources for next of kin after any death of a service member. Other military-sponsored programs include standard mental health counseling, military family life consultants, Military OneSource, chaplains, and family readiness programs. Each service also offers survivor-specific support groups. Organizations outside DoD, such as the Tragedy Assistance Program for Survivors, Gold Star Wives, and the VA, also offer support and bereavement counseling for loss survivors. It is not known whether DoD and outside organizations are providing evidence-based care consistent with research recommendations.

Respect and Honor

There is almost no literature to guide appropriate ways to respect and honor decedents or their loved ones. Resource guidelines provide procedural recommendations, such as protecting the confidentiality of suicide decedents and their loved ones. In addition, the guidelines for respecting and honoring loss survivors largely overlapped with those focused on grief support, such as the importance for organizational leaders to "reach out" to loss survivors, and conflicting evidence about holding memorial services.

In contrast, there are a large number of DoD processes and procedures for respecting and honoring the fallen, including guidelines for memorials and funeral services, posthumous awards and honors, and presidential letters of condolence for those service members who take their own lives in a combat zone. There are also legal and policy requirements regarding how next of kin are to be notified and how the body will be transported. There are a number of benefits for which loss survivors may be eligible, administered by either DoD or the VA. When suicide deaths are determined *not* to have occurred in the line of duty, loss survivors may be ineligible for certain types of benefits, as shown in Table S.1.

Table S.1
Loss Survivor Benefits, Administering Department, and Effect of LoD Determination

Benefit	Administering Department	Affected by LoD Determination
Loss survivor benefit plan	DoD	Yes
Death gratuity	DoD	No
Disbursement of pay and allowances	DoD	No
Housing allowance	DoD	No
Burial benefits	DoD	No
Dependency and indemnity compensation	VA	Yes
Servicemembers Group Life Insurance	VA	No
Dependents' Educational Assistance Program	VA	No
Burial in a national cemetery	VA	No
Identification card	DoD	No
TRICARE health and dental care	DoD	No

Perspectives of Military Suicide Loss Survivors

The military suicide loss survivors with whom we spoke made comments that centered around five themes. First, experience with CAOs or casualty assistance call officers varied. Several participants said they were paired with an officer who was caring, helpful, and knowledgeable, while other participants were paired with an officer who presumably lacked empathy and knowledge about the grief process and military administrative process. Second, loss survivors perceived administrative documents and processes, which they are encouraged to complete soon after the death, as overwhelming and challenging to navigate. Loss survivors also noted that the investigation into the details of the event was difficult to understand. Third, many loss survivors talked about being "in a fog" after their loss. They stated that grief resources and support services were challenging to navigate and too overwhelming to sort through, with one loss survivor telling us, "You don't know what you need." A fourth theme that emerged was that loss survivors felt that suicide deaths were treated differently from deaths by other means and were not given the same "honor or glory." Finally, loss survivors felt that parents and next of kin of the suicide decedent were treated differently from their spouses and that more services were needed for these other family members.

Recommendations

In light of the study results, we offer a series of 12 recommendations (presented in Table S.2) that span seven general categories:

1. Further strengthen the existing suicide surveillance system by adding elements to the DoDSER, enumerating suicide rates among members of the reserve component, and conducting in-depth investigations on suicide decedents.
2. Prepare an organizational response to suicide by developing a plan that specifies actions and responsible actors and ensures sufficient resources.
3. Work with the media to encourage factual reporting and minimize sensationalism of suicides.
4. Identify individuals at high risk.
5. Establish greater uniformity across CAOs in the ways they handle suicide deaths, consistent with standards.
6. Educate leaders, CAOs, and other support personnel about complicated grief; train health care providers on evidence-based treatments for complicated grief.
7. Reconsider whether eligibility for DoD and VA benefits should be affected by LoD determinations, and support loss survivors in making informed decisions when benefits are dispensed.

Table S.2
Study Recommendations

Recommendation Category	Recommendations
Further strengthen the existing suicide surveillance system by adding elements to the DoDSER, enumerating suicide rates among members of the reserve component, and conducting in-depth investigations on suicide decedents.	1. Incorporate fields in the DoDSER that identify data sources and the timing and severity thresholds for stressful life events. 2. Create a process to enumerate suicides among reservists and members of the National Guard not on active duty. 3. Conduct psychological autopsies on all or a sample of confirmed suicides and on a specified control group on an ongoing basis.
Prepare an organizational response to suicide by developing a plan that specifies actions and responsible actors and ensures sufficient resources.	4. Ensure that installations and military organizations are ready to respond to suicide with a detailed plan, dedicated staff responsible for implementing the plan, and sufficient resources to enact the plan. 5. Ensure that installations include in their suicide response plan a process for guiding any memorial services they conduct.
Work with the media to encourage factual reporting and minimize sensationalism of suicides.	6. View the media as a partner and encourage journalists to comply with media guidelines.
Identify individuals at high risk.	7. Implement a systematic process for identifying and referring at-risk individuals. Screening may help prevent future suicides, though there is little evidence suggesting how frequent, widespread, or extensive it should be.
Establish greater uniformity across CAOs in how they handle suicide deaths, consistent with standards.	8. Prioritize reducing variability in the quality of CAOs.
Educate leaders, CAOs, and other support personnel about the grieving process, including complicated grief; train health care providers in evidence-based treatments.	9. Make leaders and CAOs aware that grief is a normal process following death, and sudden deaths, such as those from suicide, may produce different manifestations of grief. 10. Ensure that care providers and others (e.g., military psychologists and psychiatrists, mental health providers, family counselors) who may come into contact with grieving loss survivors are aware of the symptoms of complicated grief and the cognitive behavioral approaches that have demonstrated efficacy in treating complicated grief.
Reconsider whether eligibility for DoD and VA benefits should be affected by LoD determinations, and support loss survivors in making informed decisions about benefits.	11. Consider modifying eligibility for the Survivor Benefits Plan and Dependency and Indemnity Compensation to ensure that suicide loss survivors have access to these benefits. 12. Ensure that the timing and presentation of benefits take into account loss survivors' ability to process this information in the acute period following their loss.

Acknowledgments

A number of individuals were instrumental in helping us shape and prepare this report. At the project's initiation, Ken Norton at the New Hampshire chapter of the National Alliance on Mental Illness provided sage advice and guidance. The librarians at the Suicide Prevention Resource Center, Julie Kinn at the National Center for Telehealth and Technology, and Leonard Litton in the Office of the Under Secretary of Defense for Personnel and Readiness were also helpful as we compiled our results. At RAND, Keith Jennings, Ryan Brown, Jerry Sollinger, Terri Tanielian, Sarah Meadows, and Emily Bever all provided valuable support for this research effort. We also thank our reviewers, Linda Langford and Audrey Burnam, who provided insightful and constructive feedback on this report. Our project sponsor, Captain Janet Hawkins, also provided encouragement and support throughout the course of this project.

This research effort would not have been possible without the assistance of the staff and volunteers at the Third Annual National Military Suicide Survivor Seminar and Good Grief Camp, sponsored by the Tragedy Assistance Program for Survivors (TAPS). Specifically, we are indebted to Kim Ruocco and Bonnie Carroll, both at TAPS, who supported our efforts wholeheartedly. Finally, we thank the men and women who have lost family members to suicide and agreed to share their experiences with us. Their contributions were invaluable and will inform future response efforts.

Abbreviations

AFMES	Armed Forces Medical Examiner System
ATSM	Acute Traumatic Stress Management
CACO	casualty assistance call officer
CAO	casualty assistance officer
CDC	Centers for Disease Control and Prevention
DoD	U.S. Department of Defense
DoDSER	U.S. Department of Defense Suicide Event Report
LoD	line of duty
LOSS	Local Outreach to Suicide Survivors Program
PTSD	post-traumatic stress disorder
SAMHSA	Substance Abuse and Mental Health Services Administration
SPRC	Suicide Prevention Resource Center
TAPS	Tragedy Assistance Program for Survivors
VA	U.S. Department of Veterans Affairs

CHAPTER ONE

Introduction

Background

The U.S. Department of Defense (DoD) has been struggling with increasing rates of suicide among military personnel for the past decade. Reports from a congressionally directed task force, an Army task force, and the RAND National Defense Research Institute have all made a series of recommendations to help DoD address this issue. DoD continues to implement new programs and examine its policies in an effort to prevent more military men and women from taking their own lives.

Purpose

The objective of this research was to assess DoD's response to suicides among military personnel and to identify opportunities for enhancing DoD programs and policies. This report has two purposes.

First, an earlier RAND report, *The War Within: Preventing Suicide in the U.S. Military* (Ramchand, Acosta, et al., 2011), recommended that DoD "provide formal guidance to commanders about how to respond to suicides and suicide attempts." This report reviews the scientific evidence to date, complemented by the perspectives of those most intimately touched by military suicide—the family and friends of those who have died—to help DoD formulate its guidance in a practical and efficient way.

In compiling this report and conducting the literature review, it became apparent that there is little scientific evidence about how best to respond to suicides, how to ensure that surveillance activities are managed appropriately and that loss survivors are given sufficient support to grieve,[1] how additional suicides can be prevented, and how to honor and respect the decedent and his or her loved ones. At the same time, there are many resource guides intended to provide recommendations for organizations (mostly schools) in responding to suicides. We reviewed a large number of these resource guides to identify and categorize their recommendations. We then assessed what research evidence exists to support each recommendation. The purpose of this review was to help leaders craft a coordinated response to suicide by informing them of which strategies they should prioritize adopting. In an area as emotionally wrought as suicide response, it is imperative that we not conflate emotion with science, and this report seeks to help distinguish between the two.

[1] Throughout this report, we use the phrase *loss survivors* to refer to the family and friends of a person who has taken his or her own life.

Approach

The research on responding to suicides is thin, so we drew from multiple data sources to inform our study. Specifically, data come from four sources: a review of the scientific literature, a review of DoD policies and procedures, the perspectives of loss survivors of military suicide, and an analysis of resource guides intended to help organizations respond to suicides.

We examined the evidence base according to four broad categories: suicide surveillance, preventing suicides after a suicide, grief after suicide, and respect and honor for those who die by suicide and their survivors. In each case, we reviewed the scientific evidence supporting various actions DoD could take in response to a suicide. We then examined the policies and procedures that guide how DoD currently responds to suicide. Finally, we examined how resource guides address each category and identified what evidence exists to support each recommendation.

The Evidence Base

We conducted our literature review using the PubMed, PsycInfo, and MEDLINE databases, searching on terms specific to each of the four aforementioned categories. We included only empirical studies and systematic reviews or meta-analyses. Once the articles were selected and reviewed, we examined their reference lists to identify other relevant studies that might have been missed in the initial search. The review was expressly focused on evidence supporting actions in the period after a suicide. For reviews of suicide prevention strategies, see *The War Within: Preventing Suicide in the U.S. Military* (Ramchand, Acosta, et al., 2011, chapter 3) and *Evidence-Based Suicide Prevention Strategies: An Overview* (Mann and Currier, 2011); for reviews on interventions for those at risk for suicide, see Mann, Apter, et al. (2005).

DoD Policies and Procedures

To identify DoD policies and procedures, we reviewed Titles 10 and 38 of the U.S. Code for legislation relevant to the death of a service member and, more specifically, death by suicide. We also reviewed DoD and U.S. Department of Veterans Affairs (VA) policies and guidance relevant to service member and veteran deaths, suicides, mortuary affairs, casualty assistance programs, awards and ceremonies, and burials and funerals to identify the full complement of relevant practices. Finally, we examined the services' policies on the same range of topics to identify the comprehensive policy and guidance framework that supports how they respond to suicides.

Analysis of Resource Guides

There are a number of publicly available guides that DoD leaders might draw upon to inform their response to suicide. To our understanding, however, there has been no initiative to compile the recommendations from different guides to ensure that they guidance they offer is consistent.

We reviewed and assessed multiple guides to identify the types of recommendations available using the Suicide Prevention Resource Center's (SPRC's) postvention and crisis response online library.[2] At the time of that review (December 2010), it contained 41 docu-

---

[2] Supported by the Substance Abuse and Mental Health Services Administration (SAMHSA) and operated by Education Development Center, Inc., SPRC "promotes the implementation of the National Strategy for Suicide Prevention and

ments published by such organizations as the Centers for Disease Control and Prevention (CDC), SAMHSA, and the National Association of School Psychologists. A complete list of the resource guides is presented in Appendix A.

The research team reviewed the 41 documents and extracted each unique recommendation, excluding recommendations that focused exclusively on suicide prevention and intervention. Items included in lists of directives, and paragraph titles, or headings related to postvention were considered recommendations. The team then employed a three-step strategy to produce a consolidated list:

1. We extracted and compiled all recommendations from the 41 SPRC documents and collapsed redundant recommendations, resulting in 652 unique recommendations.
2. We collapsed the 652 recommendations into 183 categories.[3] Ninety recommendations were not classified because they focused on responses to nonfatal suicide attempts (e.g., recommending counseling for the attempter and his or her family members, ensuring the physical health of attempter, maintaining ongoing contact with a counseling agency regarding treatment progress and goals), because they were ill defined or vague (e.g., envisioning a community with better or more resources, mitigating potential long-term psychological problems, reaching out), or because they applied only to school settings (e.g., asking teachers and friends about the child, preventing other students from witnessing a traumatic event, helping children understand what might happen next).
3. We employed a second stage of inductive classification by placing each of the 183 recommendations into 31 categories.[4]

We identified which of the 31 categories of recommendations related to each of four themes (surveillance, suicide prevention after a suicide, helping loss survivors grieve, and honoring and respecting those who have died by suicide and their friends and family members); recommendations could belong to more than one theme. For example, the category "Convey postvention messages strategically" was classified as relating to both preventing future suicides and helping loss survivors grieve. Most categories were classified under multiple objectives because actions often have multiple intentions. Disagreement over a category's classification was resolved via consensus. All recommendations abstracted from the resource guides and considered in this study are listed in Appendix B.

To provide a snapshot of how installations across the services currently respond to suicides, we set out to learn more about the experiences of military suicide loss survivors. This group is an understudied population, and no research to date has evaluated its needs. To conduct this qualitative assessment, RAND collaborated with the Tragedy Assistance Program for Survivors (TAPS), a national nonprofit that provides resources to individuals who have suffered the loss of a service member. We conducted focus groups with a sample of attendees at a

---

enhances the nation's mental health infrastructure" (SPRC, undated). In support of this mission, it offers an online library of resources on various topics related to suicide, including postvention.

[3] For example, the recommendations "Use various forms of communication including TV and radio" and "Identify several modes of communication for both internal and external communication" were classified under the action "Use multiple media to convey postvention messages."

[4] For example, "Use multiple media to convey postvention messages" was listed under the category "Convey postvention messages strategically" along with 13 other recommendations related to communicating messages.

national military loss survivor conference to collect information on the needs and experiences of those who have lost a service member to suicide.

Organization of This Report

The first four chapters of this report examine the science behind postvention and current DoD policies: Chapter Two addresses suicide surveillance, Chapter Three presents research and guidelines on preventing suicides in the aftermath of a suicide, Chapter Four covers grief after suicide, and Chapter Five addresses the topic of respect and honor for those who die by suicide and those they leave behind (referred to as *loss survivors*). Each chapter follows the same structure. First, we review the evidence base for each topic area and provide a description of DoD policies, procedures, and practices. We then review recommendations from resource guides on each topic, and the evidence base supporting the different categories of recommendations. We conclude with a summary of the evidence and recommendations and assess the degree to which DoD policies, practices, and procedures conform to the evidence base.

Chapter Six provides insight on the responses of loss survivors of military suicides. It provides both the unique perspectives of family and friends and an intimate snapshot showing how the military, in practice, responds to suicide deaths. Chapter Seven concludes the report by synthesizing the findings from prior chapters to provide a series of recommendations that DoD, the services, and installations might consider adopting to strengthen their current response to suicides. Two appendixes offer a list of the resource guides reviewed and a detailed overview of our review, respectively.

CHAPTER TWO

Surveillance

Suicide surveillance involves tracking and reporting information related to a suicide. A public health approach to prevention is built around surveillance because it enables "realistic problem solving, facilitates the design of prevention programs, and the ability to evaluate such programs" (Bonnie, Fulco, and Liverman, 1999). However, as discussed elsewhere (Ramchand et al., 2011; Goldsmith et al., 2002; Crosby, Ortega, and Melanson, 2011), systematic surveillance of suicide in the United States is lacking. This is largely because of variability in the degree to which suspected suicides are investigated, jurisdictional variation in the requirements for making a suicide determination, and regional differences in how equivocal deaths are classified. As discussed later, these issues are minimized for suicides among those on active duty in the armed forces but are relevant for suicide surveillance among veterans and members of the reserve component (i.e., the National Guard and reserves).

Our literature review on surveillance focused on three areas: (1) the CDC's 1988 guidance to medical examiners and coroners on making suicide determinations, (2) the CDC's 2011 uniform definitions and data on self-directed violence surveillance, (3) the utility of psychological autopsies for suicide surveillance and recently developed standards for conducting such autopsies.

The Evidence Base

Cause-of-Death Determination

There are long-standing concerns about the validity of suicide surveillance, a result of both differing assessments of those who make cause-of-death determinations and differences across jurisdictions in the policies and processes that guide death investigations. In 1988, a working group of representatives from the American Academy of Forensic Sciences, American Association of Suicidology, Association of Vital Records and Health Statistics, CDC, International Association of Coroners and Medical Examiners, National Association of Counties, National Association of Medical Examiners, and National Center for Health Statistics published operational criteria for determining suicide (Rosenberg et al., 1988), and that document remains the primary reference on the topic (Crosby, Ortega, and Melanson, 2011).

The two conditions required for determining suicide as the cause of death are that the death was self-inflicted and that "at the time of the injury the decedent intended to kill himself or herself or wished to die and that the decedent understood the probable consequences of his or her actions" (Rosenberg et al., 1988). Typically, medical examiners do not have a problem determining that an injury was self-inflicted and identifying manner of death using evidence from autopsy results (e.g., distance from which a bullet was fired), toxicology reports, investigations (police reports or crime scene photographs), or statements of the decedent or witnesses. Determining suicidal intent, however, is much more complicated. For example, the presence of drugs or alcohol or a history of mental illness could make it difficult to determine whether the decedent intended to die. The working group highlighted the following four scenarios in which it is especially difficult to determine intent:

> (1) when death is delayed or when it is the unanticipated consequences of a potentially self-destructive act; (2) when a body is never found; (3) when drownings, leaps, or falls are unwitnessed; or (4) when the death is of a child too young to realize the consequences of jumping from a window, swallowing poison, or running in front of a car. (Rosenberg et al., 1988, p. 1449)

To help medical examiners and coroners establish intent, the working group offered examples of the type of evidence that might facilitate making such a determination. Explicit evidence can include "verbal or nonverbal expression of intent" to kill oneself (Rosenberg et al., 1988). However, the group also highlighted examples of some implicit evidence, presented in Table 2.1. It is important to note that while these examples can help guide a death determination, there are many reasons, besides intent to die, that someone would engage in the behaviors

Table 2.1
Categories of Implicit Evidence of Intent to Die and Examples

Category of Implicit Evidence	Examples
Preparations for death inappropriate for or unexpected in the context of the decedent's life	Unexplained giving away of possessions or making provisions for the future care of children or pets
Expression of farewell or a desire to die or an acknowledgement of impeding death	"I won't be kicked around anymore"; "You were real important to me."
Expression of hopelessness	"It just doesn't matter anymore"; "What's the use of. . . ?"
Expression of great emotional or physical pain or distress	"This pain is killing me"; "I can't stand it anymore"; "I cannot live like this."
Effort to procure or learn about means of death or to rehearse fatal behavior	Recently purchasing firearms and ammunition
Precautions to avoid rescue	Locking doors, going to a prearranged, secluded place
Evidence that decedent recognized the high potential lethality of the means of death	Researching different drugs to determine their degree of lethality
Previous suicide attempt	Previous nonfatal attempt, including self-destructive acts carried out with the goal of killing oneself
Previous suicide threat	A statement of intent; playing with a gun and saying, "I'm going to shoot myself."
Stressful events or significant losses (actual or threatened)	Loss of a relationship, intangible losses (being passed over for promotion)
Serious depression or mental disorder	A diagnosed or undiagnosed mental disorder

SOURCE: Based on Rosenberg et al., 1988.

listed. These factors should not be viewed as reliable stand-alone signs of suicidal intent among living individuals.

Uniform Definitions and Data Elements

Surveillance of suicide includes not only enumerating the number of suicides in a population but also identifying elements that can help inform circumstances associated with the suicide that may have contributed to the act. In 2011, the CDC published the much-anticipated first version of its report *Self-Directed Violence Surveillance: Uniform Definitions and Recommended Data Elements* (Crosby, Ortega, and Melanson, 2011). The development of this report officially began in 2003, and over the next eight years included a scientific literature review, input from an expert panel, and revisions to draft definitions from external reviewers, including representatives from the military.

In the report, the CDC defines suicide as "death caused by self-directed injurious behavior with any intent to die as a result of the behavior" (Crosby, Ortega, and Melanson, 2011, p. 23). It recommends against the use of phrases *completed suicide* and *successful suicide* because both imply the achievement of a desirable outcome.

The recommended data elements proposed by the CDC represent a core set of items to be included in suicide surveillance systems. These elements are presented later in this chapter, when we compare them to the elements collected for DoD's surveillance program (see Table 2.2). The CDC stresses two important considerations. First, it acknowledges that collecting all the information it suggests in a core suicide surveillance system will likely require aggregating data in a relational database that draws on multiple sources, including death certificates, hospital records, emergency medical system records, surveys, health care records, and law enforcement records (Crosby, Ortega, and Melanson, 2011). As such, it recommends that the data source be an element in a surveillance system to identify the agency or organization that supplied the data, which, it says, "is essential in order to be able to distinguish the source of the information and the differences in definition from various sources" (Crosby, Ortega, and Melanson, 2011, p. 30). However, the CDC also cautions that "ethical and safety issues are foremost in any effort to examine self-directed violence" (Crosby, Ortega and Melanson, 2011, p. 15). Importantly, it stresses that it is imperative that systems are in place to protect the safety and privacy of the decedent and his or her family and friends. As such, when building relational databases, care should be taken to ensure that linkages can be made without jeopardizing confidentiality (e.g., by encrypting unique identifiers).

Psychological Autopsies

Because suicide is rare and it is difficult to study it using prospective epidemiologic strategies, retrospective analyses that rely on psychological autopsy represent the strongest available method for identifying the antecedents of suicide. A psychological autopsy is a systematic postmortem investigation comprising interviews with key informants (e.g., next of kin or peers of the decedent) complemented by official records (e.g., hospital or clinical case notes), when possible. Many psychological autopsy studies are case studies that do not employ a control group; however, the use of a control group provides an opportunity to employ case-control analytic methods that can be used to identify risk factors for suicide (i.e., whether a certain factor occurs more frequently or closer to the date of death in the suicide group than in the control group). For psychological autopsy studies that employ a control group, that control group may include similar individuals who are alive (e.g., living community controls; Foster et al., 1999) or individuals who died by other means (e.g., veterans who died in road traffic accidents; Farberow, Kang, and Bullman, 1990). The idea of having a deceased control group has been challenged, however (Gordis, 1982). In some cases, the control group has been another group of suicide decedents. For example, one study examined suicide decedents with cancer relative to a control group of suicide decedents with no cancer history (Henriksson et al., 1995). More than 150 psychological autopsy studies have been published in the peer-reviewed literature, and the majority are case studies with no control group (Cavanagh et al., 2003).

Newer research (Conner et al., 2011, 2012) has put forth strategies for improving the "next generation" of psychological autopsy studies. Without debate, mental illness has been the best-studied construct in psychological autopsies, and a number of diagnostic interviews have been validated when conducted with proxy respondents. In a meta-analysis of these studies, Cavanagh et al. (2003) affirmed that mental illness is the most widely studied risk factor. Across findings from case studies, 90 percent of decedents have evidence of a mental illness; studies that employ a control group show a similar proportion among cases, compared with 27 percent across control groups (Cavanagh et al., 2003). Nonetheless, to improve the assessment of mental disorders, Connor et al. (2011) advocated for the study of personality disorders. In addition, they recommended examining key features of disorders, as well as psychiatric comorbidity.

Although their meta-analysis was not restricted to mental disorders, Cavanagh et al. (2003, p. 395) wrote that studies of sociological variables—contact with service agencies and health care providers, physical ill health, adverse life events, and social isolation—were all "insufficiently studied to draw clear conclusions." This position is echoed by those who have put forth strategies to improve the next generation of psychological autopsy studies. With respect to stressful life events, Connor et al. (2011) suggested the use of standardized instruments that identify event timing (when the adverse life event occurred), the severity of an event (e.g., what defines a relationship problem), the extent to which the decedent played a role in the occurrence of the event (e.g., being fired due to performance rather than losing a job due to the organization's financial status), and how other risk factors, such as mental disorders, interact with these events to confer suicide risk. They also recommended increased attention to personality traits, medical illness and functional limitations, the availability of lethal agents, and medication.

While psychological autopsy studies, particularly those with well-defined control groups, can provide a wealth of information on the antecedents of suicide in a given population, there are serious and practical procedural issues that, while surmountable, must be considered when engaging in such studies. Of critical importance are ethical considerations when interviewing family members or peers of those who have died by suicide. For example, balance needs to be struck between allowing these proxy respondents adequate time for bereavement and conducting interviews soon enough after the event to avoid recall bias. Generally, a period of two to six months is recommended, though, when feasible, interviews should be conducted sooner rather than later (Connor et al., 2012). Additional considerations and strategies for those interested in conducting such studies are described in Conner et al. (2012).

DoD Policies and Procedures

Data on military suicides are collected through military criminal investigations, autopsies, and command-directed investigations. Data on suicides are also collected and compiled in the DoD Suicide Event Report (DoDSER) for surveillance and public health purposes. We describe each procedure in the following sections.

Criminal Investigations

Depending on the circumstances surrounding a suicide, there may be several investigations conducted by numerous agencies both within and outside the military. Section 1185 of the 1994 National Defense Authorization Act (Pub. L. 103-160, 1993) required DoD to issue a regulation requiring investigation into the deaths of service members from self-inflicted causes. In response, DoD issued an instruction titled "Investigation of Noncombat Deaths of Active Duty Members of the Armed Forces" (DoDI 5505.10, most recently reissued in 2013) directing the services to train criminal investigation officers in appropriate procedures for investigating noncombat deaths.[1] The policy also stipulated that these officers are to conduct an investigation even if a civilian organization had jurisdiction and had done a separate investigation but had not performed an autopsy. Each service has its own entity that is responsible for carrying out these investigations: There is the U.S. Army Criminal Investigation Command (comprising soldiers trained in investigation), the Air Force Office of Special Investigations (both airmen and civilian personnel), and the Naval Criminal Investigative Service (almost entirely civilian personnel).

Autopsies

All deaths of *active-duty* service members require an autopsy. Title 10, Chapter 75, of the U.S. Code directs DoD's Armed Forces Medical Examiner System (AFMES) to conduct an investigation into a death if the cause of death appeared to be unnatural or is unknown. The services all employ a medical examiner and a mental health expert (in the case of an apparent suicide) to determine whether the cause of death was suicide or some other cause. When a death does not occur on a military installation, civilian authorities conduct autopsies and the services can request to be involved in ongoing investigations. AFMES is required to provide the results of any autopsy and the decedent's remains to the next of kin as soon as practical after the completion of the investigation (DoDI 5154.30, 2003).

In 2010, the DoD Task Force on the Prevention of Suicide by Members of the Armed Forces published the results of its congressionally mandated investigation into military suicides. The task force found that AFMES performed 36.1 percent of the autopsies on suicide cases between January 1, 2003, and March 31, 2009. It also found that there were inconsistencies in civilian autopsies, conflicts between civilian and military determinations, and delays in the determination of death due to the slow speed with which civilian autopsies were completed. The task force recommended legislation that would enable a more facile transfer of autopsy information between civilian and military organizations, and, as of this writing, DoD was working with the VA to facilitate the more timely transfer of such data.

---

[1] As described in Chapter Five, the instruction also directs criminal investigation organizations to establish family liaison programs.

Line-of-Duty Investigations and Determinations

After the death of an active-duty service member, another type of command-driven formal investigation is conducted by the services, known as a line-of-duty (LoD) investigation.[2] These investigations occur after certain injuries, illnesses, or deaths and are intended to ascertain whether the event was due to negligence or misconduct on the part of the service member. One of two determinations results from an LoD investigation: The incident occurred in the line of duty, or the incident did not occur in the line of duty. In the case of a death, the determination refers to whether the death occurred during the normal conduct of duty or whether there were qualifying circumstances that made the incident *not* within the normal conduct of duty. Generally, deaths among active component service members are considered to have occurred in the line of duty. However, if the death was determined to be the result of misconduct or negligence on the part of the service member, the investigation would conclude that the death was not in the line of duty. If the death was not in the line of duty, loss survivors may not be eligible for survivor benefit retirement payouts. This issue is described in greater detail in Chapter Five.[3]

Service-specific regulatory guidance stresses that a suicide determination must be made on the basis of substantial evidence. Regulations stress that the law presumes a sane person will not choose to take his or her life or attempt to take his or her life, and, thus, by extension, a suicide is caused by temporary or permanent insanity. All instances of insanity lead to a determination of "in the line of duty," and loss survivors therefore receive all benefits. In some cases, there may be evidence that the death was not due to mental unsoundness, in which case the investigating officer must present overwhelming evidence to show soundness and therefore derive the determination of "not in the line of duty due to. . . ." In the conduct of the LoD investigation, investigating officers may ask the service member's unit about his or her behavior prior to the suicide or attempted suicide, determine whether a blood alcohol test was conducted, interview friends and family about the service member to determine whether he or she asked for help, determine whether a firearm was involved and the service member's level of expertise with that kind of firearm, and check with local authorities to determine whether a civil investigation was conducted and, if so, request the case records. The investigating officer may use any report by the criminal investigating organization as evidence in the investigation, as well as any reports produced by civilian police, coroners' offices, and medical personnel.

For suspected suicides, investigating officers are also directed to include a mental health assessment with their final determination. A mental health officer must review all the collected evidence to determine the biopsychosocial factors leading up to the suicide or attempted suicide. Based on this evidence, it is up to the mental health officer to determine whether the service member's psychological condition existed prior to service or was aggravated by service, as well as whether the service member was sane at the time of death and thus whether the suicide was due to the service member's own misconduct. Any self-inflicted disease, injury, or death that resulted from a suicide attempt by a service member considered mentally sound is considered the fault of the service member, hence the determination will be "not in the line of duty due to own misconduct." This determination will lead to a loss of benefits, as described in greater detail in Chapter Five.

---

[2] Information about LoD determinations was drawn from service-specific regulations and policies.

[3] For an example of loss survivor benefit plan characteristics, see U.S. Army, 2014.

The VA has an identical legal parameter regarding LoD determinations, which may preclude loss survivors' access to benefits administered by the VA system. In the event of a suicide, the VA will conduct its own investigation, which may produce disparate findings, leading to a different determination from the service investigation. As is the case with DoD, the VA will not determine the act to be willful misconduct if mental illness was a factor. If the person was mentally unsound and the unsoundness was related to military service, then the veteran's survivors are eligible for full VA benefits.[4]

In 2010, the DoD Task Force on the Prevention of Suicide by Members of the Armed Forces found that investigations were inadequate for informing suicide prevention programs and instead focused on potential criminal activities or cause-of-death issues. The task force recommended that DoD conduct a root-cause analysis over a two- to three-year period to determine which data elements would enhance the DoDSER, as well as to enhance understanding about suicide causality in the military (U.S. Department of Defense Task Force on the Prevention of Suicide by Members of the Armed Forces, 2010). Further, the task force recommended that family members be allowed to participate more fully in the investigative process, suggesting that the interaction between criminal investigative agencies and the decedent's family would benefit both parties (U.S. Department of Defense Task Force on the Prevention of Suicide by Members of the Armed Forces, 2010).

Surveillance, Reporting, and Information

In response to the National Defense Authorization Act for Fiscal Year 2007 (Pub. L. 109-364, 2006), DoD issued guidance to the services to record and report a full and accurate account of deceased personnel (DoDI 1300.18, 2009). Casualty reporting to the service is required within 12 hours of a death and is captured in the Defense Casualty Information Processing System. As of 2009, suicides were recorded separately in the DoDSER once AFMES had determined that the casualty was a suicide. Figure 2.1 shows this process.

The DoDSER was created to standardize suicide data collection and reporting across the services and to report qualitative information collected during investigation of a death.[5]

Figure 2.1
DoDSER Process Flowchart for Fatal Events

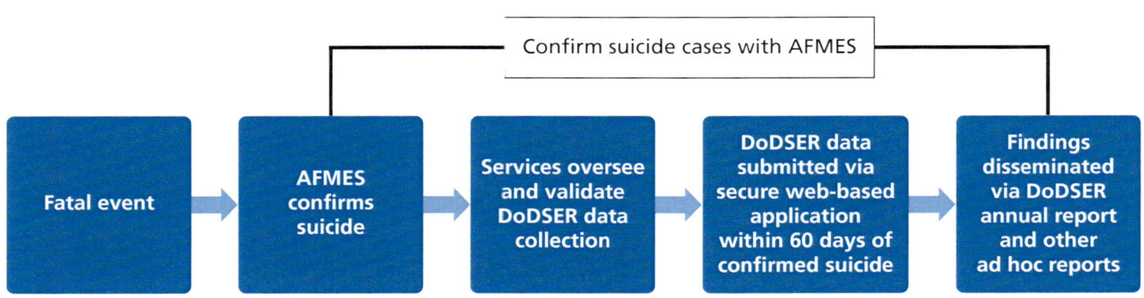

SOURCE: Adapted from Gahm et al., 2012.
RAND *RR586-2.1*

[4] For more information on willful misconduct and VA benefits, see Lawyers.com, undated. Allowances are also articulated in Title 38, Section 1110, of the U.S. Code.

[5] Also see Under Secretary of Defense for Personnel and Readiness, 2006.

The National Center for Telehealth and Technology oversees the DoDSER and the systematic tracking of suicide deaths, but, as shown in Figure 2.1, the services are individually responsible for overseeing data collection. This was a fact noted by the congressionally directed DoD Task Force on the Prevention of Suicide by Members of the Armed Forces, which reported that "standardization of the DoDSER is hindered by variable processes regarding who collects and enters data and the lack of training for the surveyor" (U.S. Department of Defense Task Force on the Prevention of Suicide by Members of the Armed Forces, 2010, p. 99).

Nonetheless, the DoDSER represents a marked improvement over the un-integrated systems of the past. It contains a variety of elements, with strong correspondence between the core data elements recommended by the CDC (see Table 2.2). Items recommended by the CDC but not contained in the DoDSER include data sources, risk rescue ratings (the degree to which the situation allowed for the possibility of intervention by others to prevent death), injury severity, previous suicidal thoughts, and sexual orientation (Gahm et al., 2012).

The DoDSER was launched in 2008. Therefore, it was relatively new when the congressionally directed task force indicated that, while it was an improvement over existing surveillance systems, the DoDSER lacked "dynamic, interview-based, observations of symptoms, behaviors, and communications along the pathway to suicide across the last days of life" (U.S. Department of Defense Task Force on the Prevention of Suicide by Members of the Armed Forces, 2010, p. 100). The task force stated that such data would greatly assist the military in understanding issues related to suicide. It also recommended that DoD conduct a case-control study using data from a separate data system, the Defense Medical Surveillance System, on matched controls to better understand military suicide causes and contexts, which the creators and DoDSER administrators agreed would "provide an extremely valuable resource for analyzing suicide risk factors" (Gahm et al., 2012).

Resource Guidelines

Our review of the postvention guides available through SPRC's online library uncovered recommendations related to surveillance that spanned eight broad categories (see Table 2.3), but they were generally focused on increasing sensitivity during cause-of death-investigations and pre-planning to ensure that organizational responses to suicides are coordinated and support surveillance activities.

Sensitivity During Cause-of-Death Investigations

The recommendations "Ensure proper documentation" and "Provide guidance for death scenes" are most directly related to surveillance. The first addresses the importance of confirming that a death is a result of suicide before treating it as such. Although cause-of-death determinations will be made almost immediately in some cases, it may take time for medical examiners to confirm equivocal cases as suicides. Ensuring the cause of death is particularly important for loss survivors, both because of the emotional toll of a suicide loss (see Chapter Four) and because the determination affects the benefits and resources for which they may be eligible (see Chapter Five). Some guidelines also stress the importance of documenting the actions and decisions made after a suicide, which could be especially useful for the organization in its self-evaluation plans and in modifying established response plans (discussed in the next section).

Table 2.2
Core Data Elements Recommended by the CDC for Suicide Surveillance and Inclusion in the DoDSER

Categories	CDC Core Data Elements	Included in the DoDSER?
Identifying information	Case ID	Yes
	Data source	No
Demographics	Sex	Yes
	Age and birth date	Yes
	Race	Yes
	Ethnicity	Yes
	Marital status	Yes
	Residence	Yes
Socioeconomic status	Education	Yes
	Occupation	Yes
	Industry or economic activity	Yes
Event information	Manner of injury (i.e., the role of human intent)	Yes
	Place of occurrence	Yes
	Date and time of injury	Yes
	Nature of injury (e.g., blood vessels, crush)	Yes
	Mechanism (how the injury was inflicted, e.g., firearm, cutting/piercing)	Yes
	Activity (what the victims was doing at the time of the incident)	Yes
	Alcohol use	Yes
	Drug use	Yes
	Severity of injury	No
	Disposition (action or status after attendance; this is used more for suicide attempts than for suicides)	Yes
	Medical care received	Yes
	Self-directed violence category (for those who die, this is either fatal suicidal self-directed violence or fatal undetermined self-directed violence)	Yes
	Suicidal thoughts at time of injury	Yes
	Risk-rescue rating ("degree to which the situation allowed for the possibility of intervention by others to prevent death")	No
Individual and family history	Previous medical history, somatic	No
	Previous medical history, mental	Yes
	Previous medical history, suicidal behavior	Yes
	Previous medical history, suicidal thoughts	No
	Previous medical history, family medical/psychiatric	Yes
	Previous medical history, sexual orientation	No
	Military service	Yes
Associated factors	Proximal factors (including precipitating events, such as recent history of personal crisis)	Yes
	Protective factors	Yes
	Incident summary	Yes

SOURCES: Crosby, Ortega, and Melanson, 2011; Gahm et al., 2012.

Table 2.3
Surveillance Recommendations Derived from Resource Guides

Type of Recommendation	Recommendation (Number in Appendix B)
Sensitivity during cause-of-death investigations	Ensure proper documentation (6)
	Provide guidance for death scenes (10)
	Interact with families appropriately (16)
Pre-planning	Create a response plan (24)
	Ensure necessary infrastructure (15)
	Establish a suicide response team (25)
	Promote collaboration between organizations (2)
	Involve senior leaders (18)

The recommendation "Provide guidance for death scenes" concerns the handling of an investigation in the immediate aftermath of a suicide. Although investigation procedures follow their own prescribed guidelines, the published guidelines recommend that those charged with death scene investigations be sensitive to witnesses and loss survivors, including not punishing individuals who may have interfered with the scene. In line with this goal and as described in Chapter Three, the Local Outreach to Suicide Survivors (LOSS) program makes crisis workers and paraprofessional volunteers available at the death scene with the goal of providing direct and immediate support to loss survivors and promoting sensitivity among investigators.

The recommendation "Interact with family members appropriately" is directed toward organizations that interact with families, stressing that organizations should proactively reach out to families to make them aware of the suicide, how the organization will respond to the suicide, and what resources are available for support. This is relevant to surveillance because, in some instances, a death may not be determined a suicide for some time, and family members may need to assist in the investigation. There are different recommendations regarding whether interactions with families should occur in writing or in person, and there is no scientific evidence to support one method over the other. As with the recommendations for death scenes, those for interacting with families generally stress sensitivity throughout the course of these communications; in Chapter Five, we discuss in more detail DoD policies and procedures for notifying next of kin after suicide deaths.

Pre-Planning

The remaining five recommendations in Table 2.3 are important for surveillance but pertain to preparations that organizations should undertake prior to a suicide. They stress the importance of (1) creating a response plan, (2) having the necessary infrastructure to respond, (3) establishing a suicide response team, (4) ensuring collaboration among organizations, and (5) ensuring strong leadership buy-in. With respect to surveillance, these recommendations are generally synergistic: Plans should be conducted and teams should be established to ensure that an organization's surveillance and investigation procedures unfold smoothly and efficiently. With respect to collaboration, this may mean ensuring that parties within the organization and in the community that are called upon to respond to a suicide death (e.g., law enforcement, departments of mental health, crisis centers) are aware of or help develop the suicide response plan and know the members of suicide response teams. Because organizations may go long periods without involvement in the aftermath of a suicide, and because team members may change, many guidelines stipulate that plans should be updated routinely. Finally, there are guidelines stressing the importance of strong leadership buy-in to help facilitate the planned response.

Conclusion

DoD's suicide surveillance efforts generally surpass those in civilian settings, particularly for active-duty personnel. For members of the National Guard and reserves, surveillance often suffers from the same issues that affect civilian suicide surveillance: variability in the degree to which suspected suicides are investigated, jurisdictional variation in the requirements for making a suicide determination, and regional differences in how equivocal deaths are classified.

The DoDSER is an important source of information about suicide deaths that can help inform characteristics and events associated with suicide. While the DoDSER has significant overlap with many of the fields that the CDC recommends, noticeably lacking is a field that identifies the source from which each data element is derived. This information is critical for establishing the validity of data and for uncovering discrepancies in aggregated data.

While the DoDSER is an important source of information for suicide surveillance, carefully constructed psychological autopsy studies can complement this surveillance system, particularly if a control group is used to compare against suicide decedents. There are two psychological autopsy studies currently under way in the Marine Corps and the Army (Ramchand, Eberhart, et al., 2014). The findings from these studies can provide rich information that can be used to guide the development of targeted suicide prevention programs.

Published guidelines rarely deal with issues specific to surveillance. One set of recommendations focuses on ensuring that loss survivors are treated with sensitivity during death-scene and subsequent investigations. The other set relates to ensuring that the appropriate infrastructure is in place to conduct surveillance and that response teams are aware of surveillance procedures. Though these recommendations lack a very strong evidence base, they align well with the goals of surveillance and can ensure that surveillance activities are conducted thoughtfully and efficiently.

CHAPTER THREE

Suicide Prevention After a Suicide

Communities affected by suicide, while bereaved, may also be motivated to use the event to reinvigorate policies, procedures, and activities designed to prevent future suicides. The occurrence of a suicide may heighten community awareness of suicide, its risk factors, and its consequences. This may then provide an opportunity for leaders to garner additional support and energy for implementing suicide prevention best practices.

A previous RAND report presented a review of suicide prevention research (Ramchand et al., 2011). Much of that report and its recommendations are relevant to this study of suicide postvention. In this chapter, we review the following particularly relevant points: (1) evidence indicating that those who experience the death of someone close are at increased risk for suicide and suicide contagion, (2) empirical support for programs or activities that are relevant to preventing future suicides, and (3) media influences on suicide. For a more detailed discussion of these and other topics, we refer readers to the reviews in *The War Within* (Ramchand, Acosta, et al., 2011), among others (e.g., Goldsmith et al., 2002; Mann et al., 2005b; van der Feltz-Cornelis et al., 2011).

The Evidence Base

Suicide Risk Among Loss Survivors

After a suicide, the decedent's surviving family, friends, and colleagues may be at heightened risk for suicide. There is evidence that those bereaved by suicide are at risk for experiencing suicidal ideation, which is associated with increased risk for mental disorders and suicidal behaviors (Beck et al., 1999; de Groot, Neeleman, et al., 2010; de Groot, de Keijser, and Neeleman, 2006). One study compared close friends and acquaintances of an adolescent who had died by suicide to a demographically matched control group that was not exposed to a suicide (Brent, Perper, et al., 1993). Although there were no differences between the groups in rates of suicidal behavior, the study did find that those exposed to suicide reported significantly higher rates of suicidal ideation, depression, and post-traumatic stress disorder (PTSD). Based on their findings, the authors recommended that organizations conduct intensive, long-term clinical follow-up assessments of psychological problems, such as depression, with friends of suicide decedents. We discuss screening programs implemented after a suicide later in this chapter, and we examine evidence-based treatments for grief-related psychological symptoms among family and friends of suicide decedents in Chapter Four.

Suicide contagion is defined as "a process by which exposure to the suicide or suicidal behavior of one or more persons influences others to commit or attempt suicide" (Gould,

Wallenstein, and Davidson, 1989). Suicide clusters are generally defined as a "group of suicides that occur closer together in time and space than would normally be expected in a community" and may include online communities (Rajagopal, 2004). While statistical approaches have been developed to help define a suicide cluster (Gibbons, Clark, and Fawcett, 1990; Cheung et al., 2013), some suggest that statistical verification (e.g., reliance on statistical significance) of a suicide cluster might miss important information that is needed to prevent future suicides (O'Carroll and Mercy, 1990). For example, perceptions of a cluster (whether statistically verified or not) within the community could lead to overestimation of the prevalence and acceptability of suicide, which could sway some individuals to attempt suicide.

Young people (e.g., adolescents) appear to be more vulnerable to suicide contagion than older age groups (Gould, Wallenstein, et al., 1990). Individuals who have been experiencing mental health problems (such as depression), those who were close to or peers of the person who died by suicide, and those exposed to heightened community and media attention, including glorification of the decedent, may be particularly susceptible to suicide contagion as well (Brent, Kerr, et al., 1989; O'Carroll, Crosby, et al., 2001; Pirkis, Blood, et al., 2006). For example, Carr (2011) describes how soldiers and mental health staff experienced increased distress following one soldier's suicide on deployment in Iraq. The author notes that existing mental health problems among some soldiers appeared to be exacerbated by the suicide, leading a few individuals to be medically evacuated and to receive intensive treatment (Carr, 2011).

Empirical Studies Examining Post-Suicide Prevention Activities

When examining research studies that evaluate the effects of a practice or intervention, it is critical to examine the quality of the study's methodology. Randomized controlled trials are intervention studies in which participants are randomly assigned to receive either the intervention (e.g., counseling, medication) or something besides the tested intervention (e.g., usual care, placebo pill, assessment only). They are the standard for quality research (Lohr, 2004). We were unable to find any randomized controlled trials that tested a program implemented after a suicide to prevent future suicides or to interrupt suicide clusters or contagion. However, suicide is a statistically rare and relatively unpredictable event, which makes planning a large, rigorous randomized controlled trial after a suicide particularly challenging.

Although there have been no randomized controlled trials, other studies have documented organizational responses to suicide (and, in some cases, compared different responses), offering insight for our study. Following two unrelated suicides within three months in two separate high schools, researchers in the United Kingdom implemented a study to compare the responses. At both schools, one group of students volunteered to receive a one-time 90-minute counseling session following the suicide, and a comparison group of students at each school received no counseling at all (Hazell and Lewin, 1993). The counseling session was conducted within seven days of the suicide and focused on the participants' understanding of what led to the suicide and personal reactions to the suicide, with the acknowledgment that some of the students in the session may have felt suicidal themselves. Participants were also made aware of the various support services available to them through the school and in the community. Students from both groups were evaluated approximately eight months after the counseling intervention to determine whether there were differences in their levels of suicidal ideation or suicidal behaviors. No differences were detected between the groups on a range of outcomes, including suicidal ideation, depression, and drug and alcohol use (Hazell and Lewin, 1993). These findings may have been influenced by characteristics of the students who received counseling: Those who self-identified as close friends of the decedent were specifically targeted to receive counseling services, though this process was found to be inefficient in that many close friends did not get referred to counseling. The findings also could have been affected by the amount of time that had passed since the suicide; students may have naturally learned to cope in the aftermath of the suicide during this time. These findings are, however, consistent with a meta-analysis showing that the prevention of complicated grief among bereaved individuals (not limited to suicide loss survivors) has not been effective (Wittouck et al., 2011; a more detailed discussion is also provided in Chapter Four).

We identified no studies specifically designed to test the interruption of suicide contagion and the prevention of suicide clusters. In light of the dearth of evidence specifically addressing how to prevent suicide clusters, in 1987, the CDC and the New Jersey Department of Health sponsored a workshop to develop recommendations for helping community leaders plan to respond to suicide clusters or situations that might lead to suicide clusters (O'Carroll, Mercy, and Steward, 1988). The working group put forth the following recommendations:

1. Review these recommendations and develop a response plan before the onset of a cluster.
2. The community's response should involve all concerned community sectors and should be coordinated by
   a. a coordinating committee (to manage day-to-day crisis response)
   b. a host agency (responsible for "housing" the plan, monitoring suicides, and calling meetings of the coordinating committee).
3. Identify relevant community resources.
4. Implement response plan either
   a. when a suicide cluster occurs in the community
   b. when one or more deaths from trauma occur in the community, especially among adolescents or young adults, which may potentially influence others to attempt or commit suicide.
5. As a first step in implementing a response plan, contact and prepare groups that will play key roles in the first days of the response.
6. Respond in a manner that avoids glorification of the suicide victim and minimizes sensationalism.
7. Identify people who may be at high risk for suicide and who have had at least one screening interview with a trained counselor; refer these individuals for further counseling or other services as needed.
8. Provide a timely flow of accurate, appropriate information to the media ("CDC Recommendations for a Community Plan for the Prevention and Containment of Suicide Clusters," 1988; the article provides more detail on these steps, which are paraphrased here).

Although these recommendations provide some guidance for communities and organizations to consider after a suicide to prevent a possible cluster, they are drawn from expert opinion, a method with the lowest level of evidence quality among tested research strategies (see Centre for Evidence Based Medicine, 2013).

Hacker and colleagues (2008) described a multifaceted intervention incorporating the CDC's recommendations that was implemented after a series of suicides and overdoses were observed in young people in Somerville, Massachusetts. The intervention involved a broad range of public and private organizations and was supported by local community leadership

(Hacker et al., 2008). Components of the intervention included the development of a surveillance system to detect suicide clusters and contagion, screening for suicide risk factors, increased availability of crisis counseling, raised awareness of and screening for suicide risk factors, cooperation with local media outlets to report suicides in accordance with established guidelines (discussed later in this chapter), and equal treatment of suicides and other deaths to avoid stigmatization. After implementing the intervention, the authors observed decreased rates of suicide and overdoses. However, the authors acknowledged that, due in part to the lack of any control or comparison condition, these positive outcomes could have been a result of other, unmeasured factors.

Recently, organizations and individuals have developed models to help guide organizational responses to suicide. Two such programs, LOSS and Connect, are described here.

Local Outreach to Suicide Survivors Program

Campbell and colleagues (2004) described an "active postvention program" that they piloted outside Baton Rouge, Louisiana, called the Local Outreach to Suicide Survivors Program (LOSS). Collaborating with local law enforcement and other first responders in the local community, crisis center workers and paraprofessional volunteer suicide loss survivors formed LOSS teams that arrived at the scene of a suspected suicide with other first responders. At the scene, the LOSS team helped comfort loss survivors, explained the investigative activities being conducted, and provided information about available community resources; the presence of paraprofessional volunteers was meant to instill hope that the loss survivors could cope with the traumatic loss (Campbell et al., 2004). The LOSS team personnel developed personal relationships with first responders and were able to gain their trust. These first responders then provided the volunteers with access to death scenes, where the volunteers could provide immediate assistance to loss survivors. In addition, the teams sensitized first responders to the needs of loss survivors.

Preliminary evidence suggests that the LOSS program has been effective in encouraging loss survivors to reach out for support at the crisis center that sponsored the LOSS teams. In 2008, Cerel and Campbell examined the efficacy of the LOSS program by comparing the recipients of LOSS support (n = 150) to loss survivors who did not participate in the program (n = 206) in terms of service utilization and problems with appetite, exercise, sleep, and concentration. There were no significant demographic differences (e.g. sex, age, race) between the two groups of loss survivors, but the decedents of LOSS participants were more likely to have died by violent means and to have a history of mental health problems or prior suicide attempts. LOSS survivors were also more likely to have discovered the decedent's body and less likely to have received a suicide note. The groups did not differ in family history of suicide or rates of their own mental health problems (including suicidal ideation) prior to the suicide. The investigators found that those who received LOSS program support were more likely to seek counseling at the Baton Rouge Crisis Intervention Center (69 percent versus 59 percent) and that they sought these services more rapidly than those who received the standard response (within an average of 48 days, compared with 97 days, respectively). However, the groups did not differ in reports of appetite, exercise, sleep, or concentration problems, suggesting that the program may not improve mental health outcomes. Further, because the decedents of LOSS participants tended to have more serious prior histories of suicidal behaviors, to have died by more violent means, and to not leave notes, it is unclear whether observed differences in outcomes were due to these preexisting differences rather than the LOSS program itself. Related to this limitation, suicide loss survivors were not randomly assigned to each condition, and it is not clear how groups were selected. More rigorous evaluation of this program is needed to determine whether LOSS is effective in improving the long-term outcomes of suicide loss survivors and whether there are other benefits—for example, whether the presence of LOSS teams helps sensitize other first responders at the death scene.

Connect

The Connect postvention program was developed by the New Hampshire chapter of the National Alliance on Mental Illness; it provides training for community members and service providers that "increases the capacity of a community or organization to respond effectively to a suicide death in order to prevent additional suicides and promote healing for survivors of suicide loss" (Suicide Prevention Resource Center, 2008). It is an ecological prevention model consisting of general training on identification and referral of individuals in distress and discipline-specific training for law enforcement officials, clergy, and others who, because of their profession, may be more likely to come into contact with a person in distress. This discipline-specific training is designed to enhance community coordination across providers who are charged with caring for individuals at risk for suicide and to ensure that all parties are aware of their role in responding to a suicide.

Connect was designed as a prevention model and was adapted to enhance communities' responses to suicides. Specifically, it seeks to improve understanding and awareness of the impact of suicide on loss survivors, ways to facilitate coping and healing after a suicide, and the identification of roles and responsibilities for service providers to take on after a suicide. There is a Connect postvention training tailored specifically to military communities.

While no published study has evaluated Connect's postvention program, studies have evaluated it as a prevention program. Specifically, two studies involved administering questionnaires both before and after the three-hour training sessions and found that the training improved participants' knowledge about suicide and beliefs in the usefulness of mental health care, reduced stigma associated with seeking help, and increased preparedness to help (Baber and Bean, 2009; Bean and Baber, 2011). More research is needed to determine whether the postvention adaptation is effective in meeting its identified goals and whether it leads to community reductions in suicide.

Insight from the General Suicide Prevention Research

Other evidence from the general suicide prevention literature is informative for the purposes of this study. In *The War Within*, RAND researchers identified the following key components of a comprehensive suicide prevention program:

1. Raise awareness and promote self-care.
2. Identify those at risk.
3. Facilitate access to quality care.
4. Deliver quality care.
5. Restrict access to lethal means.
6. Respond appropriately (Ramchand, Acosta, et al., 2011).

We discuss how identifying those at risk through screening and delivering quality care is relevant to prevention following a suicide, and we draw primarily on research that is not specific to postvention.

Screening

Screening for suicide risk can occur in a variety of venues. Most research to date has focused on school or primary care settings. Some studies have proposed that screening for suicide risk be implemented quickly and broadly following suicide incidents (O'Carroll and Mercy, 1990). Typically, screening programs identify individuals at risk for suicidal behaviors through the use of standardized screening instruments. Studies on the efficacy of screening programs in these different settings are currently under way, though existing studies have yielded inconsistent results. The efficacy of universal screening programs, in which everyone in a given group is screened for suicide risk, has been tested primarily in schools. While, to date, no screening program has been shown to reduce suicide rates, there has been some evidence that such programs yield promising effects. For example, there is some evidence that screening helps identify those who are thinking about suicide but who have not asked for help on their own (Husky et al., 2009) and who otherwise would not have been identified by school staff (Scott et al., 2009). With respect to primary care, the U.S. Preventive Services Task Force recommends that primary-care physicians screen for depression but does not provide a recommendation for or against specifically screening for suicide risk (U.S. Preventive Services Task Force, undated).

Based primarily on concerns about the risk of suicide contagion, some have hypothesized that asking youth about suicide risk in a screening program can have iatrogenic, or unintended, adverse effects or may lead to suicidal thoughts and attempts. A rigorous randomized controlled trial found no evidence that screening for suicide risk increases suicidal thoughts or behaviors (Gould, Marrocco, et al., 2005). However, for such a screening program to be effective, it is critical that adequate referral resources be available for those identified as being at increased risk (Hallfors et al., 2006).

Delivery of Quality Care

Some clinical interventions have been shown to be effective in preventing suicide among individuals with histories of suicidal thoughts and behaviors. Dialectical behavior therapy, a mental health treatment protocol that typically lasts for one year, has been shown to reduce suicide attempts among individuals with borderline personality disorder displaying suicidal or self-injurious behavior (Linehan et al., 2006). Cognitive therapy has also been shown to reduce suicide attempts among prior attempters (G. Brown et al., 2005). Even relatively low-effort interventions, such as sending "caring letters" to patients with depression, has led to reduced suicides (though replication of this model has not produced consistent results; Aoun, 1999; Morgan, Jones, and Owen, 1993; Motto and Bostrom, 2001).

There is indirect but still convincing evidence that improved depression awareness among health care professionals can lead to reductions in suicides (Rutz, von Knorring, and Walinder, 1989). Evidence-based psychotherapy and pharmacotherapy that improves mental health symptoms also might reduce suicides indirectly by improving mental health symptoms (Blue Ribbon Work Group on Suicide Prevention in the Veteran Population, 2008; Goldsmith et al., 2002; Leitner, Barr, and Hobby, 2008). Caring for those at risk for suicide occurs at many levels; thus, in addition to delivering evidence-based care, it is critically important that people have ready access to treatment and that treatment is delivered with continuity across the system of care (National Action Alliance for Suicide Prevention, 2012; Ramchand, Acosta, et al., 2011). Studies have found that many individuals had seen a mental health professional a short time before dying, but a review of these data suggests that a breakdown in the continuity of care minimized the effectiveness of the system in preventing these suicides (Luoma, Martin, and Pearson, 2002).

The delivery of quality mental health care can also include means-restriction efforts, the fifth component of the comprehensive suicide prevention strategy described in *The War Within* (Ramchand, Acosta, et al., 2011). For example, assessing individuals for suicide risk and restricting their access to lethal means, such as firearms or pills, are key elements in intervening with individuals in crisis (e.g., individuals who access crisis intervention services, suicide hotlines, and the emergency room). Protocols for assessing risk and safety planning, such as the Collaborative Assessment and Management of Suicidality (Jobes et al., 2005) and SAFE VET (Suicide Assessment and Follow-Up Engagement: Veteran Emergency Treatment; Stanley and Brown, 2008; Knox, Stanley, et al., 2012), have been developed as one way to help restrict patients' access to lethal means in hospital and employment settings. These protocols have not yet been evaluated, but there is evidence to suggest that parents of adolescent suicide attempters can be taught about means restriction by emergency department staff and that such training can encourage parents to limit their children's access to lethal means (Kruesi et al., 1999; McManus et al., 1997).

For both screening and care delivery to be effective in preventing suicide, individuals must feel comfortable accessing care. There are a number of factors that influence whether individuals seek mental health care, including their own recognition of mental health problems (Fikretoglu et al., 2008), their social network and the social support they receive from it (which can both positively and negatively influence mental health service utilization; Maulik, Eaton, and Bradshaw, 2009), and distrust of the military health and mental health systems (Fikretoglu et al., 2008). These same factors may also affect individuals' tendencies to use suicide prevention techniques, such as questioning a high-risk colleague about his or her suicidal thoughts and referring him or her to treatment (Mishara, Houle, and Lavoie, 2005).

Finally, evidence-based therapies for complicated grief (reviewed in Chapter Four) hold promise as ways to treat psychological symptoms and prevent suicide; a description of treatments for complicated grief and their level of efficacy is presented in Table 4.2 in Chapter Four (see also Wittouck et al., 2011). In addition, for the bereaved and for community members more generally, behavioral and pharmacological interventions (e.g., cognitive behavioral therapy, antidepressants) that have been shown to be effective treatments for symptoms of depression and other suicide-related risk factors may be useful.

Media Coverage of Suicide

A number of research studies have examined the influence of media coverage of suicides on actual suicide rates in the general population. Across studies, there is a general consensus that increased publicity of suicide is correlated with increased suicide rates in the community, though this effect has been demonstrated primarily among adolescents. A number of reviews and meta-analyses conclude that media coverage of celebrity suicides has a particularly strong effect and that the effect of media coverage of "authentic" suicides is stronger than the effect of fictional accounts. In addition, accounts in daily newspapers exert a larger effect than television accounts, and more balanced reporting of a suicide poses less risk than reporting that is sensationalistic, with detailed descriptions of the method of suicide or accounts of the setting

(Gould, 2001; Pirkis and Blood, 2011a, 2001b; Schmidtke and Schaller, 2000; Stack, 2005; Wasterlund, Schaller, and Schmidtke, 2009; Bohanna and Wang, 2012; Sisask and Värnik, 2012).

In response to these media effects on suicide, a number of guidelines have been published for the media on how to appropriately cover suicides. These guidelines stress avoiding what is known to increase suicide risk and aim to educate journalists that the amount, duration, and prominence of coverage relates to the rate of increased risk, that risk increases when stories explicitly describe the suicide method or use dramatic or graphic headlines or images, and that coverage that sensationalizes or glamorizes death should be avoided. The guidelines not only relay what not to do but also stress strategies to enhance proper coverage that can encourage those who are vulnerable to seek help. Explicit guidelines developed by a consortium of advocates and experts are available through reportingonsuicide.org and are presented in Table 3.1.

While many countries have established guidelines for the media on how to report on suicides, the effect of implementing these guidelines on suicide are inconclusive (Pirkis, Dare, et al., 2009; Mann, Apter, et al., 2005). The strongest evidence comes from a series of studies on the introduction of media guidelines in Austria in 1987 and the subsequent decline in the overall suicide rate. The decline was largely attributed to a reduction in subway suicides, which had increased markedly and were the impetus for creating the guidelines (Etzersdorfer and Sonneck, 1998; Etzersdorfer, Sonneck, and Nagel-Kuess, 1992; Niederkrotenthaler and Sonneck, 2007). Most other research has found that journalists are generally unaware of and do not use any particular guidelines (Bohanna and Wang, 2012) and that results are mixed about whether the publication of guidelines leads to sustained changes in media reporting on suicides

Table 3.1
Guidelines for Responsible Reporting of Suicides in the Media

Instead of This	Do This
Big or sensationalistic headlines, or prominent placement (e.g., "Kurt Cobain Used Shotgun to Commit Suicide")	Inform the audience without sensationalizing the suicide and minimize prominence (e.g., "Kurt Cobain Dead at 27").
Including photos/videos of the location or method of death, grieving family, friends, memorials, or funerals	Use a school/work or family photo; include hotline logo or local crisis phone numbers.
Describing recent suicides as an "epidemic," "skyrocketing," or other strong terms	Carefully investigate the most recent CDC data and use non-sensational words like "rise" or "higher."
Describing a suicide as inexplicable or "without warning"	Most, but not all, people who die by suicide exhibit warning signs. Include the "Warning Signs" and "What to Do" (from reportingonsuicide.org) in your article, if possible.
"John Doe left a suicide note saying. . . ."	"A note from the deceased was found and is being reviewed by the medical examiner."
Investigating and reporting on suicide in a manner similar to reporting on crimes	Report on suicide as a public health issue.
Quoting/interviewing police or first responders about the causes of suicide	Seek advice from suicide prevention experts.
Referring to suicide as "successful," "unsuccessful," or a "failed attempt"	Describe as "died by suicide" or "completed" or "killed him/herself."

SOURCE: Recommendations for Reporting on Suicide, undated.

(Sisask and Värnik, 2012). In a review of 240 different military and civilian newspaper reports of suicide from 15 different sources, Edwards-Stewart and colleagues (2011) found that only one article fully adhered to SPRC's media guidelines. The authors also found that military and civilian articles differed in style: Civilian reports tended to romanticize the decedent, whereas military reports more frequently used negative language to describe the decedent and referred to ineffective behavioral health treatment as a contributor to the suicide (Edwards-Stewart et al., 2011).

While experts create guidelines and public health organizations around the world advocate their use, it should also be noted that there has been some empirical evidence that the introduction of these guidelines has increased reporting of suicides, and, when introduced with strong and comprehensive dissemination efforts, content did adhere more closely to the guidelines (Fu and Yip, 2008; Michel et al., 2000; Pirkis, Dare, et al., 2009). In addition, another recent Austrian study found that newspaper stories that focused on suicide research, provided information about a public support service, and reported expert opinions—which some guidelines recommend—were actually associated with an increased suicide rate, though these articles also may have included statements that societal problems are increasing, which some deem problematic (Niederkrotenthaler, Voracek, et al., 2010).

DoD Policies and Procedures

There is currently no DoD-wide policy or guidance that directs or suggests that commanders implement suicide prevention trainings or perform on-site investigations to identify possible suicide clusters or strategies for intervening if one suspects that a cluster is forming immediately following a suicide. Similarly, although the services and suborganizations may have their own media guidelines, there are no official DoD-sponsored guidelines for reporting on or discussing suicide with the media.

However, there are at least three types of responses that the services have adopted as a result of an increase in suicides. First, in at least two instances the services have revised or revamped their approach to suicide prevention. Second, they have held stand-downs to focus service-level attention on suicide prevention. Third, they have evaluated their approach to suicide prevention. In many instances, these responses have overlapped.

Revising Prevention Programs

From 1990 to 1994, suicide rates in the Air Force increased enough that senior leaders made suicide prevention a priority. Drawing from 15 different functional areas, the Chief of Staff of the Air Force directed a study that produced 11 initiatives to strengthen social support, promote coping skills, and change policies and norms to encourage help-seeking. The Air Force Suicide Prevention Program was deemed at least partially responsible for a decrease in suicide rates between 1997 and 2002. As suicide rates rose again in the early to mid-2000s the Air Force significantly revamped its program, as described in the following section (see Knox et al., 2003).

The 1996 suicide of the Navy's most senior officer, Chief of Naval Operations Admiral Jeremy Michael Boorda, increased awareness of suicide among sailors. Although Admiral Boorda's suicide was perhaps not the singular cause (1991–1996 was a period of escalating suicide rates in the Navy), in 1998, the Navy instituted a new behavioral health program.

Stand-Downs

In 2009, the Army ordered a one-day service-wide stand-down in response to elevated rates of suicide (Headquarters, U.S. Department of the Army, 2009), and certain posts, such as Fort Carson, Colorado, took more than a day to address especially concerning trends (Hall, 2009). The Army order directed its units to conduct suicide prevention training in three phases for all soldiers, Army civilian staff, and family members to "increase awareness of suicide risk factors and warning signs and to encourage intervention for at risk soldiers" (Headquarters, U.S. Department of the Army, 2009). The stand-down was the first phase of the three-phase intervention, with one day of suicide prevention training between February 15 and March 15, 2009, and included all U.S. Army Reserve and National Guard units.

Similarly, in May 2010, the Air Force Chief of Staff and Chief Master Sergeant of the Air Force directed a half-day stand-down to address elevated rates of suicide and motor vehicle accidents. Rate of suicide in the service had steadily increased since 2007, and the Air Force stand-down included a half-day training on suicide prevention and coping skills to improve psychological resilience (Russell P. Petcoff, 2010). Although it was not formally evaluated, the Wingman Day stand-down was considered by Air Force leaders to be so successful that the Chief of Staff of the Air Force instituted a two-day period every year to address total fitness, team-building, and other resiliency activities. In fact, the Air Force suicide prevention strategy shifted in 2010 to focus more on improving the total fitness of Air Force personnel and established the Resiliency Division within Air Force headquarters to focus on airman and family resilience (Jones, 2011).

Evaluations of Existing Programs

In 2008, with increasing rates of military suicide causing significant concern, Congress directed DoD to establish a task force to examine ways to prevent suicide and report recommendations for a comprehensive policy to prevent suicide, with one year to complete the initiative (Pub. L. 110-417, 2008, Section 733). Ultimately, the task force reported 76 major findings across four areas: organization and leadership, wellness enhancement and training, access to and delivery of quality care, and surveillance, investigations, and research.

In addition to the congressionally directed task force, DoD and the services sponsored comprehensive evaluations of their own suicide prevention programs. For example, DoD commissioned a RAND report that resulted in 16 recommendations (Ramchand, Acosta, et al., 2011), and the Army continues to conduct its own evaluations (see Headquarters, U.S. Department of the Army, 2010, 2012).

Resource Guidelines

Overall, we identified 18 categories of recommendations related to preventing suicide in the resource guides we examined (see Table 3.2). They generally dealt with pre-planning to respond to a suicide, identifying individuals at high risk of taking their own lives after the event, communicating with the media and loss survivors, and using the moment to revise or rejuvenate suicide prevention programs.

Table 3.2
Suicide Prevention Recommendations Derived from Resource Guides

Type of Recommendation	Recommendation (Number in Appendix B)
Pre-planning	Ensure necessary infrastructure (15)
	Create a response plan (24)
	Establish a suicide response team (25)
	Ensure resources are available (26)
	Promote collaborations between organizations (2)
	Foster a supportive community (8)
Identifying high-risk individuals	Conduct gatekeeper training (9)
	Monitor community members and resources (22)
	Screen for high risk individuals (28)
Communication	Convey postvention messages strategically (12)
	Interact with the media strategically (17)
	Do not use inappropriate words, terms, and images in communications (20)
	Use appropriate words, terms, and images in communications (21)
	Provide guidelines for leaders (11)
	Conduct appropriate memorial services (19)
Using, reviewing, and rejuvenating suicide prevention training	Conduct suicide prevention training (29)
	Conduct an environmental risk assessment (7)
	Enforce rules and restrictions (27)

Pre-Planning

The recommendations related to infrastructure and creating a response plan are generally consistent with the CDC guidelines for the creation of a community response to interrupt suicide clusters described earlier (see the section "Empirical Studies Examining Post-Suicide Prevention Activities"). Although some of the recommendations in these areas are general (e.g., "Respond in a timely manner") and might not provide valuable guidance above and beyond the CDC guidelines,[1] others are more specific (e.g., "Develop a process to handle donations") and could augment the CDC guidelines in the formation of a plan. Collectively, these recommendations represent a relatively comprehensive list of potential components of a response plan.

Identifying High-Risk Individuals

Three categories related to preventing future suicides by focusing on strategies to identify vulnerable individuals after a suicide death. In this domain, the recommendations stress that (1) support staff should receive gatekeeper training, (2) organizations should monitor high-risk groups, and (3) formal screening procedures should be established to identify individuals at high risk. While more informal recommendations for gatekeeper training and informal moni-

[1] A full list of recommendations can be found in Appendix B.

toring may be important, there is no evidence that these strategies reduce suicide or encourage referrals or help-seeking after a suicide (Ramchand, Ayer, et al., forthcoming). Furthermore, past research—conducted primarily in schools—has stressed that universal screening approaches are better at identifying individuals at high risk than those that rely on informal referrals (Scott et al., 2009). There is also evidence that school staff and faculty are unable to identify all individuals who might benefit from mental health services after a suicide (Hazell and Lewin, 1993).

Communication

Communication guidelines focus on what messages should be delivered and how. Consistent with the research literature suggesting that certain media presentations of suicide can lead to contagion, one category of recommendations included guidelines on interacting with the media that were generally consistent with research suggesting that organizations treat the media as a collaborative partner (Langford, Litts, and Pearson, 2013) and include the media in any organizational response plan. It is also recommended that organizations encourage media outlets to follow guidelines for reporting on suicide; some of the resource guides we reviewed even provide their own guidelines about what to say and what not to say, many (but not all) of which overlap with the reporting guidelines on suicide (Recommendations for Reporting on Suicide, undated). However, some recommendations may conflict with others. For example, one set of guidelines recommended that organizations avoid blaming the victim, while others recommended that they convey that the victim is responsible for his or her actions. Depending on how the guidelines are presented and interpreted, they could be seen as leading responders in opposite directions. One group of recommendations encouraged publishing available resources. While this seems sensible and adheres to the media guidelines, it is important to note that one study found that publishing this material in newspapers was associated with increases in suicide, though these articles tended to also include statements about increasing rates of suicide that some would deem problematic (Niederkrotenthaler, Voracek, et al., 2010).

The resource guides often translate the media guidelines for reporting on suicide to how suicide should be discussed with members of the decedent's organization or community. These recommendations may stress the importance of using several outlets to convey messages, but some suggest a letter while others suggest small-group formats. Many guidelines recommend having a script prepared in advance. Again, while many of these recommendations derive from studies on contagion and the impact of media reporting, there is no evidence to suggest that one strategy has more merit than another.

There were also recommendations about the importance of memorials and how to conduct them (e.g., "Focus memorials on how to prevent future suicides"). There were conflicting recommendations in this category as well. For instance, one recommendation was "Conduct on-campus memorial services," while another stated, "Do not conduct on-campus memorial services." Again, there is a general absence of research guidance on these issues. Thus, research findings on the media and avoiding the glorification of suicide deaths offer the strongest evidence available on these topics.

Using, Reviewing, and Rejuvenating Suicide Prevention Training

Finally, three groups of recommendations suggest very specific activities in which organizations can engage after a suicide to prevent subsequent suicides. First, there is a series of recommendations to establish or re-offer suicide prevention training after a suicide. This may refer to targeted, discipline-specific training or more general training, consistent with the aforementioned Connect suicide postvention model (Baber and Bean, 2009; Bean and Baber, 2011). Two other groups of recommendations, on the other hand, stress preventing suicide by modifying the environment. Some guidelines recommend that organizations conduct an "environmental risk assessment" to identify what elements may contribute to suicide in the environment (i.e., the availability of lethal means or absence of safeguards, such as fences on bridges) and ultimately change them. This guideline is in accordance with research suggesting that reducing access to lethal means is an effective suicide prevention strategy and should be adopted when possible. On the other hand, guidelines specific to schools that recommend not permitting individuals to leave the campus may be unrealistic to enforce on military installations and could foster anger and frustration among those whose movement is restricted.

Conclusion

A suicide may heighten the risk of suicide among those close to the decedent or other potentially vulnerable people within an organization. There is evidence of suicide contagion and suicide clusters, including in the U.S. military (Associated Press, 2008; Goode, 2009; Hourani, Warrack, and Coben, 1999). Similarly, there is a relationship between media coverage of celebrity suicides and suicide rates; however, no study has investigated the relationship between media coverage of military suicides and changes in the military suicide rate.

These factors suggest that strategies should be implemented after a suicide to prevent subsequent suicides. However, there is little scientific research to suggest *what* exactly should be done. The strongest evidence is based on expert consensus, included in the CDC guidelines that are now more than 20 years old regarding how communities might prevent suicide clusters, as well as more recent expert consensus on media guidelines for reporting on suicide. Recommendations from the resource guides specific to preventing suicide after a suicide often derive from what is known about media coverage of suicide and emphasize avoiding the overglorification of suicide deaths or the decedent.

The postvention guidelines we reviewed also offer some unique suggestions and some evidence of effectiveness, though not specific to postvention. For example, some recommendations suggest screening for high-risk individuals, and there is some empirical support for this. In addition, environmental risk assessments can identify environmental factors that can be modified to reduce the likelihood of subsequent suicides. Also consistent is that strategies to respond should be thought out and planned in advance.

DoD practices are generally reactive to an increasing trend: Broad-level evaluations of prevention efforts are conducted, approaches to suicide prevention are reformulated, and the services or suborganizations conduct stand-downs. There is no guidance or protocol for suborganizations or installations to follow after a single suicide death to prevent subsequent suicides, so there is no way to map whether current approaches reflect the state of the art, though there is also limited evidence to even identify what the state of the art entails.

CHAPTER FOUR

Helping Loss Survivors Grieve

Intense feelings of grief are an expected, normal response to the loss of a loved one. Grief often begins with feelings of disbelief, followed by yearning, anger, depression, and, finally, acceptance (Maciejewski et al., 2007). Disbelief, yearning, anger, and depression generally peak within the first six months following the death and then begin to decline. Acceptance generally increases over the course of the first six months and continues to increase with time (Maciejewski et al., 2007). There is no firm evidence that the loss of a loved one to suicide leads to a unique clinical form of grief (Brown et al., 2007; Sveen and Walby, 2008), but a sudden or unexpected death more generally might result in particularly intense or prolonged grief reactions among family and friends of the decedent. In Chapter Six, we present the perspectives of family members and friends of military personnel who have died by suicide.

To identify the methods that most effectively help suicide loss survivors grieve, we reviewed two different but overlapping literatures: (1) research on the prevention and treatment of complicated grief and (2) research on interventions specifically designed for suicide loss survivors.

The Evidence Base

Preventing and Treating Complicated Grief

Regardless of the mode of death, research has shown that some individuals develop mental health problems, such as depression or "complicated grief" following the death of a loved one (Horowitz et al., 1997). *Complicated grief* occurs when the "typical" grieving process is seriously disrupted or stalled. It is defined as experiencing symptoms that include memories, thoughts, or images of the deceased that interfere with one's daily functioning; the avoidance of reminders of the deceased (e.g., people, places); and difficulty regaining a sense of purpose or experiencing positive emotions for longer than six months following the death of a loved one (Maciejewski et al., 2007; Shear, 2010). Complicated grief is not currently listed as a disorder in the fifth edition of the *Diagnostic and Statistical Manual of Mental Disorders* (DSM-V); however, some mental health professionals believe it should be. Between 7 and 25 percent of bereaved individuals experience complicated grief (Kersting et al., 2007; Newson et al., 2011; Shear, McLaughlin, et al., 2011; Shear, Simon, et al., 2011).

Shear (2010) outlines the following clinical features of complicated grief:

> Acute grief symptoms that persist for more than six months following the death of a loved one, including:

- Feelings of intense yearning or longing for the person who died—missing the person so much it's hard to care about anything else;
- Preoccupying memories, thoughts or images of the deceased person, that may be wanted or unwanted, that interfere with the ability to engage in meaningful activities or relationships with significant others; may include compulsively seeking proximity to the deceased person through pictures, keepsakes, possessions or other items associated with the loved one;
- Recurrent painful emotions related to the death, such as deep relentless sadness, guilt, envy, bitterness or anger, that are difficult to control;
- Avoidance of situations, people or places that trigger painful emotions or preoccupying thoughts related to the death;
- Difficulty restoring the capacity for meaningful positive emotions through a sense of purpose in life or through satisfaction, joy or happiness in activities or relationships with others.

We began our review of the literature on the prevention and treatment of complicated grief by examining a meta-analysis on the subject (Wittouck et al., 2011).[1] Wittouck et al. examined findings from 14 randomized controlled trials of complicated grief prevention and intervention programs published between 1990 and 2007. The primary goal was to determine whether the prevention and intervention programs led to decreased complicated grief symptoms among participants. Most of the studies included samples of individuals who lost a loved one to sudden or violent means, including suicide; none focused on military populations.

Nine of the 14 studies focused on preventing complicated grief after a death using such techniques as family-based cognitive behavioral therapy (e.g., de Groot, de Keijser, et al., 2007), support groups (e.g., Goodkin et al., 1999), and writing activities (e.g., O'Connor et al., 2003). Although some studies showed small effects, the meta-analysis determined that, overall, these efforts were ineffective in *preventing* complicated grief. In other words, there is no evidence to date showing that an intervention can prevent individuals from developing complicated grief after a death. Two additional studies conducted after the aforementioned review (Sandler et al., 2010; van der Houwen et al., 2010) had disparate findings. Sandler and colleagues (2010) reported that the treatment condition (family-based cognitive behavioral group therapy) yielded greater decreases in problematic grief symptoms among youth bereaved by a parental death than among recipients of the control condition. The other study (van der Houwen et al., 2010) revealed no significant differences between the intervention (an Internet-based writing activity) and control groups on grief outcomes.

On the other hand, programs that *intervened and treated* individuals who had already developed complicated grief had positive effects overall, with participants in the interventions generally showing decreased symptoms post-treatment and at later follow-up assessments. Three of the five studies that focused on treating complicated grief incorporated cognitive behavioral interventions (Boelen et al., 2007; Shear, Frank, et al., 2005; Wagner, Knaevelsrud, and Maercker, 2006), and the other two implemented an interpretive group-based treatment (Piper, McCallum, et al., 2001; Piper, Ogrodniczuk, et al., 2007). Table 4.1 provides a brief description of the five studies that tested interventions for complicated grief. It is noteworthy that all three of the cognitive behavioral therapies yielded significant improvements in

---

1 We focus on complicated grief here because bereavement is a normal process following any sudden loss and because there are empirically supported treatments for complicated grief.

Table 4.1
Treatments for Complicated Grief

Source	Brief Description of Treatment	Demonstrated Efficacy
Boelen et al., 2007	12 weekly 45-minute individual cognitive behavioral sessions led by trained therapists following a set protocol	Therapy led to greater improvements in complicated grief symptoms compared with supportive counseling
Piper, McCallum, et al., 2001	12 weekly 90-minute sessions of group interpretive therapy led by experienced therapists	There were no significant differences in complicated grief symptoms between the interpretive therapy group and the supportive therapy group
Piper et al., 2007	12 weekly 90-minute sessions of group interpretive therapy led by experienced therapists	There were no significant differences in complicated grief symptoms between the interpretive therapy group and the supportive therapy group
Shear, Frank, et al., 2005	16 weekly sessions of individual complicated grief treatment (cognitive behavioral therapy plus components from interpersonal therapy) delivered by an experienced licensed therapist	Patients in the complicated grief treatment improved faster than those receiving interpersonal psychotherapy. A greater proportion of complicated grief treatment participants improved compared with those receiving interpersonal psychotherapy
Wagner, Knaevelsrud, and Maercker, 2006	Internet-based cognitive behavioral therapy conducted by trained psychologists and involving two weekly 45-minute writing assignments	Participants in the treatment condition showed significantly more improvement in symptoms compared with those in the waitlist control group.

complicated grief symptoms compared with control groups. The two studies testing a more psychodynamically oriented "interpretive" therapy indicated that while individuals improved over the course of treatment, treatment and control groups showed no significant differences. This suggests that cognitive behavioral approaches currently hold the most promise for treating complicated grief.

Although none of the aforementioned studies tested these interventions in populations bereaved by the suicide of a military service member, similar cognitive behavioral interventions, such as those targeting depression and PTSD, have been shown to be effective in both civilian and military populations (e.g., Tuerk et al., 2011). In addition, there is substantial overlap between cognitive behavioral complicated grief treatment and cognitive behavioral treatment for depression and PTSD and between complicated grief symptoms and symptoms of PTSD and depression. Therefore, the complicated grief treatments described in Table 4.1 are likely effective for those bereaved by the suicide of a service member as well.

Grief-Focused Support for Suicide Loss Survivors (Not Specific to Complicated Grief)

Two systematic reviews of grief-focused resources for suicide loss survivors were part of our literature search: One reviewed studies evaluating interventions for suicide loss survivors (McDaid et al., 2008); the other focused specifically on online resources for people bereaved by suicide (Krysinska and Andriessen, 2010). Neither of these reviews specifically focused on complicated grief. Instead, they focused on bereavement more generally, including typical, uncomplicated grief. We did not identify any additional empirical studies not already included in one of the aforementioned reviews or in the previously described article on complicated grief interventions (i.e., Wittouck et al., 2011).

The first (McDaid et al., 2008) reviewed eight empirical studies of interventions for people bereaved by suicide. None of the studies specifically examined treatment effects among loss survivors of military suicide. Overall, the authors concluded that substantial methodological problems in the literature inhibited their ability to draw firm conclusions about the efficacy of interventions for people bereaved by suicide. For example, only four of the studies claimed to be randomized controlled trials, and two of the four appeared not to have actually randomly assigned individuals to groups. However, McDaid and colleagues (2008) stated that, while additional research using stronger methods is critical, there is preliminary evidence that suicide loss survivors could benefit from interventions.

The content of the interventions evaluated in the eight studies varied widely, and some did not describe the intervention clearly enough to allow a full understanding of its content. In addition, the treatment targets varied widely. For example, one study (Campbell et al., 2004) evaluated an outreach program that aimed to prevent mental health problems and suicide among loss survivors by sending volunteers to death scenes to meet with them and provide support and information about resources (the LOSS program, described in more detail in Chapter Three). Another study implemented a group-based treatment centered on theories about attachment, loss, and cognitive coping for children bereaved by parental suicide (Pfeffer et al., 2002). The goal of the study was to reduce distress (symptoms of anxiety and depression) among bereaved children. In the most methodologically rigorous study reviewed, de Groot and colleagues (2007) tested whether a four-session family-based cognitive behavioral intervention would prevent symptoms of complicated grief in families bereaved by the suicide of a loved one.

The second review article examined the quality of web-based resources for suicide loss survivors (Krysinska and Andriessen, 2010). The authors identified 145 distinct websites but further evaluated only the 15 sites most frequently retrieved across various popular Internet search engines. None of the 15 sites was specifically designed for loss survivors of military suicide, and it is not clear whether any of the other 130 distinct sites were designed for this group. Eight of the top 15 sites were personal sites (i.e., designed and maintained by an individual, not an organization) devoted to suicide bereavement. Five were sites created by suicide prevention or crisis intervention organizations or programs. One was Amazon.com, the online bookstore. None of the top 15 sites was run by a national or regional organization devoted to bereavement or suicide loss survivor support.

The authors reported that, overall, the majority of the sites provided information about suicide bereavement, referral information, resources (such as suggested reading), and links to other related websites. Some of the sites provided an opportunity for visitors to interact (e.g., through discussion boards) with other loss survivors. However, because few of the sites were authored by professional, credible organizations, their overall trustworthiness is unknown. The authors also noted that most referral information directed users to loss survivor support groups and not to services delivered by mental health or other (e.g., medical) professionals. While peer support may be a helpful way to address grief after a suicide, the interventions with the most empirical support are those delivered by mental health professionals. Krysinska and Andriessen (2010) did not evaluate the efficacy of the online resources they identified in their review.

DoD Policies and Procedures

The services DoD offers to loss survivors to help them grieve almost exclusively target family members and next of kin, not fellow service members. The most common resources are casualty assistance officers (CAOs) who work with next of kin after a death and programs, offered by the military and nonmilitary organizations, that offer support for bereaved individuals.

Casualty Assistance Officers

The same policy that established the DoD suicide surveillance system (described in Chapter Two) also established responsibility within DoD for the assignment, training, and duties of CAOs (DoDI 1300.18, 2009).[2] The intent of the policy was for each service to establish a central casualty assistance office that would serve as a focal point for all casualty matters. Further, the services were to record and report on casualties accurately and in a timely fashion and be responsive to assigned CAOs.

The same instruction also stipulates the requirements for assigning CAOs, the training parameters for CAOs, and CAO duties. Table 4.2 reviews these requirements.

Military-Sponsored Programs for Military Families and Next of Kin

Myriad official DoD programs have been established to assist military dependents and colleagues with grieving and loss, though none specifically addresses loss survivor needs after a suicide. It is important to provide support for those closest to the decedent, especially his or her children, who are at substantially higher risk of dying by suicide themselves as a result of their parent's suicide (Kuramoto et al., 2013). Mental health and counseling services are available to all active-duty military personnel and their dependents, as are religious, financial, and legal services. A military family life consultant is available to work with the surviving family and is integrated with the military health system, TRICARE, and military medical facilities to ensure seamless care (see MHN Government Services, undated). Military OneSource is available to all active-duty service members and their families, as well as to reserve component service members and their families when the reservist returns from a deployment. Military OneSource offers a host of services across the range of military experiences, including dealing with credit issues, moving, and contending with the loss of a loved one. Military OneSource counselors are available in person, by telephone, and online. They are able to provide counseling services on a range of issues that may arise after the death of a service member, from grief counseling to financial and benefit counseling. Military chaplains in most major faiths are also available to both active and reserve service members and families to assist in coping with the death of a service member. All the services also have a legal assistance program, which can assist family members and loss survivors with consumer and economic issues, wills and estates, and family and domestic matters.

Each service offers a family readiness program. Family readiness initiatives and loss survivor support services are among the programs that can help family, colleagues, and friends of the suicide decedent cope with their loss. The offerings vary by military branch. Army families receive services through family readiness groups. According to Army Regulation 600-20

---

[2] We use the label *casualty assistance officers* in this report, though we recognize that each service has a different title for this role: casualty assistance officer in the Army, casualty assistance representative in the Air Force, and casualty assistance call officer (CACO) in the Navy, Marine Corps, and Coast Guard.

Table 4.2
CAO Assignment, Training Parameters, and Duties as Specified in DoD Instruction 1300.18

Category	DoDI 1300.18 Requirements
Assignment	CAO should have grade of E-6 or above.
	CAO should not be a close relative or friend of deceased.
	CAO should not be scheduled for deployment, reassignment, retirement, or release from active duty within six months.
	Casualty assistance duty must be the CAO's primary responsibility.
Training parameters	Familiarization with benefit forms and their preparation, as well as contact information for relevant agencies
	Grief and trauma awareness
	Privacy act requirements
	Public affairs practices as they relate to deceased service members and their next of kin
Duties	Provide next of kin a "DoD Survivor's Guide" booklet and a business card with contact information for a 24-hour call center.
	Assist family members with obtaining new identification cards.
	Provide next of kin with information about ongoing investigations, if applicable, and assist with obtaining a copy of those investigations.
	Assist with obtaining autopsy records, if applicable.
	Assist with obtaining legal assistance from the military, if required.
	Assist next of kin and loss survivors until all benefits have been applied for and received.
	Attend the funeral if in the local area or coordinate for another CAO to attend if in another region.
	Assist with travel and expenses for next of kin to attend the dignified transfer at Dover Air Force Base, as well as to the funeral and any military memorial. Participate in the notification process.

(2012, p. 47), family readiness groups are one of several resources designed to provide mutual reinforcement" to "Soldiers, civilian employees, retirees (regardless of marital status), and their Family members—both immediate and extended." The Navy's Fleet and Family Support Program serves the families of naval personnel. According to OPNAV Instruction 1754.1B (2007, p. 2), its centers "provide comprehensive information, programs, and referral services" to service members and their families and are operated by the Commander, Navy Installations Command. Relevant offerings include emergency preparedness and response, personal and family wellness education and counseling, and crisis intervention and response. Air Force Instruction 36-3009 (2013) establishes rules for airman and family readiness center operations, including instructions to collaborate with the installation Integrated Delivery System to "offer proactive and preventive services that promote self-sufficiency, sustain the personal and family readiness of the total force," and meet a range of other criteria (p. 4). There are 87 such centers around the world. The Unit, Personal and Family Readiness Program serves families of marines. According to Marine Corps Order 1754.9 (2012), the program's mission is to assist Marine Corps families in coping with the death of a loved one. All these service-level family readiness groups can provide support and assistance to suicide loss survivors.

Each service also has loss survivor–specific support groups. The Army's Family and Morale, Welfare and Recreation Command oversees the Army's loss survivor outreach services. Its mission is to serve as a "comprehensive network of quality support and leisure services that enhances the lives of Soldiers, Civilians, Families, military retirees and other eligible participants" (U.S. Army Family and Morale, Welfare and Recreation Command, undated).

The Navy and Marine Corps have signed agreements with TAPS, which provides peer-based emotional support; community-based care to assist loss survivors in finding support systems; assistance in resolving bureaucratic, financial, or legal problems; and a call center (Suich, 2011). The Air Force's Families of the Fallen Support Branch aims to ensure that the families of "fallen Airmen are never forgotten by providing immediate and long-term compassionate support" (Air Force Mortuary Operations, undated). This group runs the Air Force Families Forever program, which helps families maintain ongoing contact with and assistance from the Air Force.

Nonmilitary Programs for Military Families and Next of Kin

Some nonmilitary organizations also provide support. Examples include TAPS and Gold Star Wives. The VA also offers bereavement counseling for families of deceased service members. Most or all of these supporting organizations are available to active-duty service members' next of kin and loss survivors. Some of the benefits are also available to reserve service members' next of kin and loss survivors, depending on the duty status of the reservist.

Resource Guidelines

Overall, the recommendations relevant to helping loss survivors grieve reflect an emphasis on the roles of treatment providers; however, there were some guidelines on communication, identifying persons at high risk, and pre-planning that are similar to those presented in Chapters Two and Three. These guidelines are shown in Table 4.3.

Guidelines for Counselors and Other Support Personnel

The largest category of recommendations concerned what to say to loss survivors; these recommendations were directed toward counselors and other support personnel and included both general and specific guidance for how to interact with survivors (see Appendix B for a complete list). In addition, the category on preparing counselors generally emphasized the need to recognize that reactions to death by suicide vary. In aggregate, these recommendations are consistent with literature showing that there is variability in how individuals process grief and that this variability can be influenced by such characteristics as race, culture, and religion (Klass, 1999; Neeleman, Wessely, and Lewis, 1998; Rosenblatt, 2001).

There is also guidance suggesting that care providers should take care of their own individual well-being. Research evidence suggests that mental health, medical, and other care providers who hear numerous, detailed accounts of violent and tragic events can experience compassion fatigue, and some develop mental health problems (Cieslak et al., 2013; Collins and Long, 2003; Davidson and Foster, 1995; Sabin-Farrell and Turpin, 2003). The research is inconclusive on how best to prevent compassion fatigue and serious emotional distress among care providers (Eagle, Creel, and Alexandrov, 2012; Keene et al., 2010; Meadors and Lamson, 2008). However, some studies indicate that specialized training in treating bereaved or traumatized individuals, strong coping skills, and social support could buffer care providers against the development of mental health problems (Baird and Jenkins, 2003; Brockhouse et al., 2011).

Table 4.3
Recommendations for Helping Loss Survivors Grieve Derived from Resource Guides

Type of Recommendation	Recommendation (Number in Appendix B)
Guidelines for counselors and other support personnel	Use appropriate language with loss survivors (31)
	Prepare counselors (30)
	Care for care providers (1)
Communication	Provide guidelines for leaders (11)
	Interact with family members appropriately (16)
	Allow loss survivors to convene (13)
	Convey postvention messages strategically (12)
	Do not use inappropriate words, terms, and images in communications (20)
	Use appropriate words, terms, and images in communications (21)
	Promote cultural sensitivity (5)
	Protect loss survivors' privacy (23)
	Ensure confidentiality (3)
	Create groups, places, and spaces (4)
	Encourage funeral/service participation (14)
	Conduct appropriate memorial services (19)
Identifying high-risk individuals	Monitor community members and resources (22)
Pre-planning	Foster a supportive community (8)
	Provide guidance for death scenes (10)
	Ensure necessary infrastructure (15)
	Ensure resources are available (26)
	Promote collaborations between organizations (2)

Communication

Another series of recommendations provided guidance for organizational leaders as they communicate about the suicide. Specific to grief support, recommendations encouraged organizations to "reach out" to loss survivors. There was also guidance about how leaders should communicate about a suicide death with loss survivors, as well as how to convene members of the community or organization after a suicide. Instructions here generally stressed that approaches and scripts be planned in advance and encouraged flexible, multifaceted approaches: Organizations should provide resources that allow loss survivors to grieve alone or convene with others according to their individual needs, and messages should be delivered via multiple methods (e.g., in writing, in-person in a small-group setting). There is no research evidence to suggest that one strategy has more merit than another, however.

There were also recommendations regarding what organization leaders should say to those who are grieving, as well as how the media should cover suicide. While there is evidence to suggest that certain types of suicide coverage may influence contagion (see Chapter Three), there is no evidence that certain coverage prolongs or exacerbates grieving. However, adhering to media guidelines may be the best way to communicate with loss survivors in a supportive way. For example, although there is no evidence that the phrases *committing suicide* or *suicide victim* lead to contagion, exacerbate grief, or are insulting, media guidelines cite them as phrases to avoid, as loss survivors may take offense because of religious or criminal connotations. There were other recommendations for organizations to inform loss survivors of their processes and procedures for responding to a death, along with available support resources. Recommendations across the guides were consistent in suggesting that messaging should not oversimplify the suicide or its causes and consequences, should not be judgmental, and should not assign blame for not preventing the death.

There were also recommendations about the importance of ensuring loss survivors' privacy in interactions with external organizations, including the media. Though it is a topic of much debate, there is no existing research literature suggesting best practices for how to protect confidentiality following a suicide while communicating about the death with the media or the public. However, there is some literature from the fields of law and psychology that discusses these confidentiality issues (Baker, 2005; Werth, Burke, and Bardash, 2002). For example, they advise considering the potential positive and negative consequences of releasing a decedent's confidential records, including medical records, and taking into account the laws about releasing such materials. Although there are currently no evidence-based guidelines, articles discussing and highlighting these important issues could be referenced when designing confidentiality procedures (Baker, 2005; Werth, Burke, and Bardash, 2002).

Finally, there were recommendations related to memorial services and funerals. Some sources noted the importance of encouraging attendance at funerals and that having memorials provides an opportunity for loss survivors to support each other in their grief. However, recommendations about the content of such memorials often conflicted. For instance, one recommendation was "Conduct on-campus memorial services," and another source stated, "Do not conduct on-campus memorial services." Again, organizations should carefully consider the benefits and costs of following some of these conflicting recommendations in light of their particular context, as there is a general absence of outside (research) guidance on these issues.

Identifying High-Risk Individuals

Some guidelines recommended that, as in the case of suicide prevention, organizations monitor individuals who may be particularly prone to complicated grief or disruptive bereavement. To date, there is no evidence confirming the effectiveness of screening, either informal or formal, for individuals who show these symptoms. However, it may be important to ensure that all health care providers and other support personnel are aware of the symptoms of complicated grief, and provider training in recognizing mental health problems has been effective in other contexts, including suicide prevention (Mann, Apter, et al., 2005; Rutz, von Knorring, and Walinder, 1989).

Pre-Planning

Finally, recommendations also pertained to more general organizational issues, such as how to prepare for suicides. These recommendations were generally consistent with the pre-planning recommendations discussed in Chapters Two and Three, but here it is also recommended that organizations develop procedures to minimize the disruption of normal activities following a suicide. This may be important both to respect individuals' unique ways of dealing with grief (Klass, 1999; Neeleman, Wessely, and Lewis, 1998; Rosenblatt, 2001) and to avoid glorifying the suicide.

Conclusion

According to our review of the research literature, there is very little evidence for how best to support grieving suicide loss survivors or how programs can prevent complicated grief. In addition, bereaved suicide loss survivors should be aware that online resources may be unregulated and should consider that the information provided may not be reliable or evidence-based. However, for suicide loss survivors suffering from complicated grief, there is relatively strong evidence for the efficacy of cognitive behavioral interventions delivered by trained mental health professionals.

DoD and nonmilitary organizations offer many resources for those who need grief support following a service member's suicide, including CAOs, support groups, and professional mental health treatment. The effectiveness of many of these resources (e.g., CAOs) is unknown, and evaluation of these programs is needed. However, DoD mental health professionals trained in evidence-based, grief-focused interventions (such as cognitive behavioral models) can be an excellent resource for bereaved loss survivors with symptoms of complicated grief.

Published guidelines related to helping loss survivors grieve centered on training and care for counselors and others attending to bereaved loss survivors, communication about the suicide, and the planning of memorial services and funerals. (These topics are also discussed in Chapter Five.) The guidelines suggested that counselors and other professionals be sensitive to individual differences in bereavement, attend to their own mental health needs, and receive proper training and support to deliver grief-focused interventions. Guidelines suggested that when communicating about suicide, the information provided be factual and not sensationalized or overly detailed. They also recommended flexibility with the ways in which information about a suicide is communicated (e.g., depending on the audience or mode of communication) and that providers show a willingness to accommodate individual preferences and needs with regard to the grieving process. While these guidelines are potentially very useful for military leaders and those who interact with grieving loss survivors, it is important to note that more research is needed to determine whether taking such actions will help or hinder bereavement.

CHAPTER FIVE

Honor and Respect

Ensuring that a service member who has died by suicide and his or her loved ones are both honored and respected is a multifaceted process. For the fallen, it includes how the remains of the deceased are handled and arrangements for memorial services, funeral rites, or posthumous honors received. For loss survivors, it includes both practical and social challenges related to understanding the death and learning to carry on without their loved one (Cerel, Jordan, and Duberstein, 2008). Despite the importance of these activities, the scholarly literature regarding how to ensure that those who die by suicide and their loved ones are both respected and honored is limited, even though loss survivor support programs are becoming more prevalent and diverse (Cerel, Padgett, et al., 2009; Andriessen et al., 2007), and researchers are paying more attention to loss survivors' perspectives (Cutcliffe and Ball, 2009).

The Evidence Base

Respect and Honor for the Fallen

We identified only two studies relevant to respecting and honoring those who die by suicide, both of which gauged the effect of posthumous efforts on suicide loss survivors or the broader community networks surrounding the decedent. The first of these examined loss survivor responses to authorities' treatment of the bodies of decedents of traumatic deaths in the United Kingdom (Chapple and Ziebland, 2010). In their study of 80 narrative interviews, the authors found that loss survivors appreciated the opportunity to view the body. Although this activity might be "shocking or distressing," some interviewees liked having the chance to ensure that their loved one was "being cared for." The second study, a case report (Hsiung, 2007), evaluated the impact of efforts by an Internet forum moderator to respect and honor a member of the forum who died by suicide. The study found that loss survivors avoided contagion and "gradually moved on" through efforts that included a memorial page. The author observed that this page functioned as a "virtual cemetery."

These studies on modes of respecting and honoring loss survivors of traumatic deaths affirm the importance of providing opportunities for loss survivors to grieve publicly and recognize the decedent. However, the dearth of evidence precludes consensus statements regarding the appropriate handling of memorial services, funeral rites, or posthumous honors.

Also relevant is the literature on how suicide is perceived by decedents' family and friends, as well as the community more broadly. Investigations have probed how attitudes and perceptions about suicide differ. Types of suicide-related perceptions, or attitudes, assessed often include acceptability (e.g., whether suicide is justified, brave, or cowardly), one's own knowledge of suicide, and beliefs that suicide is due to poor social functioning, personal weakness, or mental health problems, such as depression or hopelessness.[1] Cultural and religious differences regarding the acceptability of suicide have been documented, though most studies have compared attitudes about suicide between and not within nations (see Colucci and Martin, 2007). More research is needed to adequately describe attitudes toward suicide within particular cultures and communities in the United States.

Respect and Honor for Loss Survivors

Two recent studies, by Dyregrov (2011) and Jordan and McIntosh (2011), reviewed the literature on loss survivors' needs following a suicide. Dyregrov (2011) found six studies that directly asked suicide loss survivors about their perceived needs (Dyregrov, 2002; Grad et al., 2004; de Groot, de Keijser, and Neeleman, 2006; McMenamy, Jordan, and Mitchell, 2008; Provini, Everett, and Pfeffer, 2000; Wilson, 2010). Jordan and McIntosh (2011) reported on five published studies (Dyregrov, 2002; Feigelman et al., 2008; de Groot, de Keijser, and Neeleman, 2006; McMenamy, Jordan, and Mitchell, 2008; Provini, Everett, and Pfeffer, 2000) and one unpublished study (see Mitchell, 2005).

Dyregrov's review concluded that suicide loss survivors' self-reported needs include help from several sources. In particular, loss survivors want support from peers who have experienced a similar loss. They also want to receive "caring" gestures from family, friends, colleagues, and others in their social network, as well as "early and outreach assistance" from professional care providers. Beyond support from others, according to Dyregrov (2011), the reviewed studies report that loss survivors need informational resources regarding the medical aspects of suicide and the grief process; help with existential, practical, economic, and legal concerns; and support for bereaved children. Finally, loss survivors want long-term follow-up care. We were unable to find guidance from the research literature on the optimal ways to deliver these types of services.

Jordan and McIntosh (2011) offer similar findings. They state that suicide loss survivors are a "significantly distressed population" that appreciates both professional assistance and interactions with others who have had a relative or close associate die by suicide. Further, according to the authors, "one size does not fit all" in terms of services for suicide loss survivors. They recommend making "multiple points of access to multiple types of services" available on a long-term basis, throughout loss survivors' grieving processes.

The overlapping results from these literature reviews show how different groups of loss survivors, representing a variety of cultural backgrounds, report similar needs. These groups included adults related to suicide decedents (de Groot, de Keijser, and Neeleman, 2006; Provini, Everett, and Pfeffer, 2000), parents of suicide decedents (Dyregrov, 2002; Feigelman et al., 2008), and adults bereaved by a suicide or natural death (Grad et al., 2004; McMenamy, Jordan, and Mitchell, 2008; Mitchell, 2005; Wilson, 2010). Therefore, while cultural and religious values, beliefs, and traditions should be considered when planning memorial services and other methods for respecting and honoring loss survivors, the research literature does provide some guidance about the most pressing needs of loss survivors across cultures and backgrounds.

These findings have several limitations, however. First, most of the loss survivors surveyed were solicited by means of convenience samples of existing support groups (i.e., those who had

[1] For a more detailed review of measures of suicide-related attitudes, see Kodaka et al., 2011.

already sought help). Thus, the studies and findings may not be generalizable to all suicide loss survivors. Second, it is not yet known how the needs of loss survivors of military suicides, in particular, might align with those of the groups investigated in these studies. In addition, the studies compared countries, whereas DoD is likely more interested in the needs of various subpopulations within the United States (e.g., parents or spouses of fallen U.S. service members). Unfortunately, there is a lack of available research to address these issues.

DoD Policies and Procedures

To respect and honor suicide decedents, the military has in place policies and procedures that describe the memorial and funeral offerings available to military personnel, as well as awards and honors that they are eligible to receive posthumously. Finally, there is a relatively new policy on presidential letters of condolence (White House, 2011).

Congress has also passed several pieces of legislation requiring DoD to create a policy that addresses the needs of loss survivors, including notification of a death, burial arrangements, and assistance in applying for benefits from DoD, the VA, and the Social Security Administration. In this section, we describe the full range of legal and policy requirements relating to the death of a service member. Then, we discuss the implications of a suicide for benefit eligibility.

Memorials and Funerals

DoD policy does not prescribe that commanders conduct a ceremony or memorial for deceased service members. At the request of the decedent's family, DoD may provide a funeral honors detail, consisting of at least one member of the individual's service. The honor involves, at a minimum, a flag presentation and the playing of "Taps."

The DoD Task Force on the Prevention of Suicide by Members of the Armed Forces found inconsistency in how DoD handles suicide memorials for deceased service members, with some installations holding memorials and others not. The task force recommended a consistent policy in DoD to address this issue and made a case that the death of a service member from suicide should not stymie the honoring of the decedent's life and service (U.S. Department of Defense Task Force on the Prevention of Suicide by Members of the Armed Forces, 2010). It is unclear to what extent efforts are being made to enforce more systematic and equitable memorial services.

Posthumous Awards and Honors

Awards may be posthumously presented to a service member's family, and a service member may be posthumously promoted, commissioned, or warranted.

Presidential Memorial Certificates and Letters of Condolence

The VA administers the Presidential Memorial Certificate program under Title 38, Section 112, of the U.S. Code; an engraved paper certificate is issued with the President's signature to honor the memory of any honorably discharged veteran. The decedent's family also receives a condolence letter from the President. In July 2011, President Obama adjusted the policy for these condolence letters, and the White House now issues condolence letters to service members who take their own lives *in a combat zone*, which previously had not been the case. In his statement, the President acknowledged the importance of honoring service to the nation and removing the stigma surrounding suicide.

Legal and Policy Requirements Relating to the Death of a Service Member

Congress has directed that DoD address the full spectrum of needs of a decedent's next of kin and loss survivors. Specifically, the U.S. Code now specifies DoD's responsibilities in the following five areas:

- identification of decedents and notification of the next of kin
- transportation and disposition of the remains of decedents, including autopsy
- provision of benefits and entitlement assistance to the next of kin and loss survivors
- liaison with the VA and the Social Security Administration
- selection and training of CAOs and data collection regarding the services they provide.

Congress has also authorized DoD to pay for all expenses associated with the transportation of the body and funeral arrangements for the deceased service member, as well as certain benefits and entitlements.[2]

The definition of *next of kin* is established by Title 10 of the U.S. Code and refers to the loss survivors who will be notified of the death and who may direct the disposition of the remains of a decedent.[3] Technically, next of kin are those who are notified, and this is established by law. The service member may designate a "person authorized to direct disposition" of his or her remains. Generally, however, this person is also officially notified in the event of the service member's death. Thus, in this report, *next of kin* includes this designee, and *loss survivors* refers to those related to or otherwise close to the decedent who were selected to receive benefits. Those eligible for loss survivor benefits and those who receive the service member's personal effects may be loss survivors *other than* next of kin.

In 2007, Congress mandated that DoD issue guidance to the services directing uniform reporting, recording, notifying, and assisting next of kin and survivors of a military decedent. Accordingly, DoD issued an instruction in 2008 stipulating

- that casualty procedures be uniform across the services, except where custom would dictate otherwise
- how the services should identify a service member's next of kin
- that these next of kin be notified promptly "in a dignified, professional, and understanding manner"

---

[2] National Defense Authorization Acts for fiscal years 2004, 2005, and 2007 (Pub. L. 108-136, 108-375, and 109-364) directed DoD to create policies for the notification of the next of kin; the act for fiscal year 2006 (Pub. L. 109-163) directed it to create policies on the transportation and disposition of remains; assistance with benefits and entitlements from DoD, the VA, and the Social Security Administration; and the selection and training of CAOs. Title 10, Section 1482, of the U.S. Code states that DoD should pay the expenses for recovery and identification of remains, notification of next of kin, preparation for burial or cremation, a casket or urn and hearse service, funeral directors' services, transportation of the remains and an escort, interment, and presentation of a flag. Title 10, Section 75, directs DoD on issues related to deceased military personnel.

[3] *Next of kin* is defined as follows: (1) the surviving spouse of the decedent, (2) blood relatives of the decedent, (3) adoptive relatives of the decedent, or (4) a person standing in loco parentis to the decedent (Pub. L. 109-364, 2006, Section 566.)

- that the decedent's remains be recovered, identified, and returned to the family expeditiously and with dignity and respect of the decedent
- that the remains be continuously escorted by a uniformed member of the services
- that the services record and release a full and accurate account of deceased or missing personnel and avoid notifying the media until 24 hours after notifying the next of kin
- that the transfer of remains at Dover Air Force Base not be made public unless approved by the next of kin and that filming of family members at Dover is not allowed
- That, in the event of an investigation, a service member's next of kin would be informed on all matters related to the investigation (DoDI 1300.18, 2009).

In turn, each service has issued policy guidance that mirrors the DoD instruction, with small differences to accommodate service customs and traditions.[4]

The Process of Notifying Next of Kin

Generally, each service's policy regulates the rank of the CAO and the notification officer (or the person who will notify the next of kin of the death, if that person is different from the CAO). Relatively senior-ranking personnel are called for, and specific uniforms and timelines have been established within each service policy on how the next of kin are to be notified. For example, all the services require next of kin to be notified within 24 hours of the death.

Service policies describe the notification of a service member's next of kin as a first step following a death, along with internal service reporting on the casualty and the initiation of investigations. After a personal visit by a member of the service, a commander will follow up with a condolence call, a letter of condolence, or both. All services treat these communications as a notification of death. Some service policies recommend specific language to use during the notification (e.g., the Navy policy recommends, "when appropriate, state that '[he or she] did not suffer'")(Navy Military Personnel Manual 1770-140, 2002). Once notification has been made, service policies stipulate that the release of information to the media should be delayed for 24 hours, in accordance with DoD guidance. All service policies state that the privacy of the service member's next of kin and survivors must be maintained, though the death essentially extinguishes the privacy rights of the decedent. The services generally recommend the use of a public affairs office to handle media requests and statements and that units offer public affairs services to loss survivors and next of kin.

The second step is generally described as assisting the family with retrieving the decedent's remains and personal effects, assisting the family with travel to the dignified transfer at Dover Air Force Base (if desired), coordinating with the funeral home for the arrival of the remains, and, if appropriate, reviewing the uniform if the decedent is to be presented dressed in a service uniform. CAOs are also tasked with, if requested, arranging for military honors at the burial and arranging for the next of kin to travel to the burial. The services pay for the transportation of the next of kin to the burial, along with the casket or urn, burial or interment expenses, and a military headstone. Honors at the burial involve the presentation of a

---

[4] The following regulations provide detailed descriptions of how each service handles a death: Army Regulation 600-8-1, 2008; Army Regulation 638-2, 2000; U.S. Department of the Army Pamphlet 600-24, 2010, (particularly chapter 4, "Postvention"); Army Regulation 600-8-4, 2008; Air Force Instruction 36-2910, 2010; Air Force Instruction 36-3002, 2012; the Navy Military Personnel Manual 1770 series, on casualty and loss survivor assistance; the Navy's *Manual of the Judge Advocate General* (U.S. Department of the Navy, Office of the Judge Advocate General, 2004); guidance from U.S. Marine Corps Manpower and Reserve Affairs (undated); and Marine Corps Order 3040.4, 2011.

flag to a next of kin. Services also allow, at the discretion of the unit commander, payment for the next of kin or loss survivors to attend a memorial service at a site other than the burial or funeral (e.g., a military memorial). Emergency financial assistance is provided at this time, and the death gratuity is processed. All service policies stipulate that the remains of deceased service members will be escorted during transit by a military officer until reaching a designated funeral home.

The third step is assisting the family in applying for and receiving benefits from DoD and other agencies. This step involves retrieving a death certificate and assisting loss survivors and next of kin in reviewing the results of any investigations and autopsies completed by the military. The key person in this chain of events is the CAO (though, again, each service has a different name for this role). The CAO is the go-between and serves the needs of the family with respect to navigating the service bureaucracies. DoDI 1300.18 (2009) lists the requirements for assigning CAOs, training parameters, and duties, which are listed in Table 4.2 in Chapter Four.

After each contact with the family, service policies require CAOs to file a full report with the service's central casualty assistance office. CAOs are also expected to access resources and get information from this office to relay to the family.

Loss Survivor Benefits

After a service member dies, the loss survivors (meaning those designated by the service member to receive benefits) can be eligible for a significant array of benefits, ranging from lump-sum payments to lifetime annuities. We describe some of the most important benefits in the following sections. It is important to note that these benefits are granted by either DoD or the VA and that eligibility for some of them is affected by the LoD determination (described in Chapter Two), as shown Table 5.1.

Table 5.1
Loss Survivor Benefits, Administering Department, and Whether They Are Affected by LoD Determination

Benefit	Administering Department	Affected by LoD Determination
Loss survivor benefit plan	DoD	Yes
Death gratuity	DoD	No
Disbursement of pay and allowances	DoD	No
Housing allowance	DoD	No
Burial benefits	DoD	No
Dependency and indemnity compensation	VA	Yes
Servicemembers Group Life Insurance	VA	No
Survivors' and Dependents' Educational Assistance Program	VA	No
Burial in a national cemetery	VA	No
Identification card	DoD	No
TRICARE health and dental care	DoD	No

There are other benefits available to loss survivors that we do not cover in this report, such as federal tax abatement, Social Security benefits, health insurance through the TRICARE system,[5] commissary and post exchange privileges, financial counseling, VA home loans, transition assistance, and bereavement counseling. None of these benefits is affected by the determination of suicide as the cause of death.

CAOs and private support organizations, such as TAPS, help families determine their eligibility and navigate the application processes. CAOs also provide a link between the family and resources provided by the service, such as public affairs officers who can assist in handling media queries and mortuary affairs officers who can assist with funeral and burial issues.

Benefits Affected by the Line-of-Duty Investigation Determination

Loss Survivor Benefit Plan

The U.S. Code establishes a loss survivor's benefit plan that grants dependents an annuity to be paid in perpetuity that is a portion of the service member's final retirement pay. In 2002, the National Defense Authorization Act amended the code to grant loss survivor benefit pay for any active or reserve component members who die in the line of duty while on active duty. Previously, if a reserve component service member died while on active duty but was not yet drawing retirement pay, his or her survivors would not receive any annuity, even if the service member had served past the initial point of eligibility (or, generally, 20 years of service). In the event of a suicide, it may be that loss survivors would not receive the loss survivor benefit plan pay if the LoD determination was "not in the line of duty."[6]

Dependency and Indemnity Compensation

Dependency and indemnity payments may be authorized for surviving families of service members who die from a disease or injury that occurred or was aggravated while on active duty, or a disease or injury incurred while in the line of duty or while on inactive duty training for reservists. The amount paid is not based on the service member's pay grade; rather, it is determined by the number of dependents, their income, and their living arrangements. There is a non–service-connected death pension for which loss survivors may be eligible as an alternative.

Benefits Not Affected by the Line-of-Duty Investigation Determination

Death Gratuity

The death gratuity is a one-time, nontaxable payment administered by DoD to assist surviving family members in coping with financial hardships caused by the loss of a service member. Loss survivors receive a payment of $100,000 if the death occurs while the service member is on active duty (or, in the case of a reservist, on inactive duty training status, active duty, or annual training or traveling to or from any of those duty statuses), or any person entering the service. There is also a lump sum gratuity of $12,420 if a service member dies within 120 days of retiring from active duty or any of the previously mentioned reserve duty statuses, but only

---

[5] Under current rules, survivors of active-duty service members who die while on active duty are eligible to receive TRICARE Prime (the military health insurance program) and the TRICARE dental plan for up to three years following the death. After the three-year period, loss survivors are eligible for the same care offered to retirees through the TRICARE system. For more detailed information about this, see TRICARE, 2014.

[6] For more information, see MyArmyBenefits, 2014.

if the VA determines that the death was caused by an illness or injury that occurred while on active duty.

Disbursement of Pay and Allowances

All pay and allowances owed to the service member at the time of death are paid to a designated beneficiary or legal representative. This means that upon the death of an active-duty service member, all owed pay, allowances, accrued leave, accrued housing allowance, travel and per diem funds, and unpaid balances of reenlistment or other bonuses are paid (DoD, 2012).

Housing Allowance

Survivors of deceased active-duty service members are entitled to 365 days of housing allowance or may remain in government quarters for up to 365 days at no charge.

Burial Benefits

DoD will care for, transport, and bury the service member, and the surviving spouse, children, siblings, and parents of the service member and of the service member's spouse are authorized to receive travel entitlements to the funeral. Travel entitlements include round-trip transportation and two days of per diem.

Survivors' and Dependents' Educational Assistance Program

A veterans' education death benefit is paid to survivors of a deceased service member.

Servicemembers Group Life Insurance

Unless a service member specifically did not choose to elect coverage, all members are covered by a VA-purchased life insurance policy. The maximum amount of coverage is $400,000 and is nontaxable. Payment is made in either a lump sum or in 36 equal installments. This insurance includes traumatic injury protection, which provides a monthly premium of $1,000 for cases of specific traumatic injury. Intentionally self-inflicted injuries are not eligible for a traumatic injury payout.

Burial in a National Cemetery

Any service member who dies while on active duty is eligible for burial in Arlington National Cemetery and in other national cemeteries, depending on local rules.

Resource Guidelines

The resource guidelines addressing respect and honor generally overlapped with those for surveillance and helping loss survivors grieve. There were a total of 16 categories of recommendations, presented in Table 5.2. Like the literature and DoD policies, these recommendations can be grouped into the categories respect for the fallen and respect for loss survivors.

Respect for the Fallen

Recommendations for respecting the fallen were largely procedural and included guidance to encourage sensitivity at death scenes, to respect the service member's culture and traditions, and to protect his or her confidentiality. There are different cultural traditions for responding to death (Metcalf and Huntington, 1991), and it is important that they be respected while surveillance procedures are conducted. As stated in Chapter Four, there is no existing research

Table 5.2
Recommendations on Respect and Honor Derived from Resource Guides

Type of Recommendation	Recommendation (Number in Appendix B)
Respect for the fallen	Provide guidance for death scenes (10)
	Ensure proper documentation (6)
	Promote cultural sensitivity (5)
	Ensure confidentiality (3)
Respect and honor for loss survivors	Prepare counselors and other support personnel (30)
	Interact with family members appropriately (16)
	Use appropriate language with loss survivors (31)
	Do not use inappropriate words, terms, and images in communications (20)
	Use appropriate words, terms, and images in communications (21)
	Provide guidelines for leaders (11)
	Care for care providers (1)
	Allow loss survivors to convene (13)
	Encourage funeral/service participation (14)
	Conduct appropriate memorial services (19)
	Protect loss survivors' privacy (23)
	Foster a supportive community (8)

literature suggesting best practices protecting confidentiality following a suicide, though law and psychology literature does discuss these issues (Baker, 2005; Werth, Burke, and Bardash, 2002).

Respect and Honor for Loss Survivors

There was heavy overlap between recommendations to help facilitate respect and honor for loss survivors and those related to helping loss survivors grieve, presented in Chapter Four. As with guidance offered to help loss survivors grieve, many of the recommendations relevant to respecting and honoring loss survivors consisted of advice to counselors and other support personnel. However, whereas for grief, guidance was given on how counselors and other support personnel should communicate with loss survivors, the relevant domains here were more general. For example, support personnel were encouraged to prepare for various responses to suicide, be sensitive to cultural traditions, and ensure that those providing care were appropriately cared for themselves.

Other overlapping categories included recommendations stressing the importance of organizational leaders "reaching out" to loss survivors, as well as guidance about how to convene and communicate with members of a community after a suicide. Again, instructions generally advocated that approaches be planned in advance and be multifaceted and flexible, though there is no research evidence to suggest that one strategy has more merit over another. Also important are recommendations about what to say; here, adhering to media guidelines may not only prevent subsequent suicides, but it could also help sensitize organizations and leaders to loss survivors' needs. Again, avoiding such phrases as *committing suicide* or *suicide victim* is a gesture of respect to loss survivors who take offense to them because of religious or criminal connotations.

With respect to memorial services and funerals, some recommendations stressed the importance of encouraging attendance at funerals. Given conflicting guidelines about how such services should be conducted and the lack of research guidance on these issues, it remains important for organizations to consider the benefits and costs of following some of these conflicting recommendations.

Conclusion

There is very little research identifying the best ways to respect and honor those who die by suicide and their survivors. In general, the research support stresses the importance of recognizing diversity: how loss survivors perceive suicide—and how they perceive death more broadly—may be influenced to a large degree by culture and tradition.

DoD has an array of policies and procedures addressing death by suicide that can serve as a way to respect and honor the fallen and those they leave behind. Topics range from posthumous awards and honors bestowed upon the deceased to burial rites and tokens of appreciation and support (such as presidential letters of condolence and financial or housing benefits).

DoD policy also addresses interactions with a service member's family and the media after a death. Methods include condolence outreach from a commander (via phone, letter, or both), and some services provide guidance about recommended language. Service policies stipulate that the release of information to the media should be delayed for 24 hours, that the privacy of next of kin and loss survivors must be maintained (death essentially extinguishes the privacy rights of the decedent), and that a public affairs office should handle media queries and be available to the service member's next of kin. These recommendations are generally consistent with those in the available published guidelines.

CHAPTER SIX

Loss Survivors' Perspectives

The impact of a suicide on next of kin or loss survivors is immeasurable and profound. Compared with loss survivors of other types of death, suicide loss survivors in the general population often report higher levels of shame, rejection, stigma, and blaming (Sveen and Walby, 2008). Loss survivors often feel stigma because their loved one died by suicide, and this often leads to social isolation, more difficult bereavement, and barriers to help-seeking (Cvinar, 2005; Jordan, 2001; McMenamy, Jordan, and Mitchell, 2008). More loss survivors report needing psychological services than the numbers who access it (Saarinen et al., 1999). Loss survivors have also expressed a need for help for their children and relief from other family stressors (Dyregrov, 2002; Provini, Everett, and Pfeffer, 2000).

Military suicide loss survivors are an understudied population. To date, no studies have evaluated the needs of this group (DoDI, 1300.18, 2009). To fulfill our stated aim to provide a snapshot of how installations across the services currently respond to suicides, we set out to learn more about the experiences of military suicide loss survivors. Specifically, we conducted a qualitative study assessing the needs and experiences of military suicide loss survivors through focus groups at a national military loss survivor conference.

Methods

Setting

RAND collaborated with TAPS, a national nonprofit organization that provides resources to individuals who have suffered the loss of a service member. Programs offered to loss survivors include peer support mentors, seminars, crisis intervention, education, and seminars and grief camps. The sessions were held at the third annual TAPS National Military Suicide Survivor Seminar and Good Grief Camp for Young Survivors in Colorado Springs, Colorado. About 177 adult loss survivors attended the camp. A total of 135 of 153 (88 percent) of adults on whom we had data experienced their loss within the previous five years. Of this group, about 47 percent were parents, 25 percent were spouses or partners, and 13 percent were siblings.

Procedures

All procedures were approved by RAND's internal review board. As attendees registered onsite at the camp, conference staff invited them to visit RAND's table to learn more about the study. RAND study team members described the focus groups as an opportunity to share recommendations about how DoD could improve its programs and policies after a service member's suicide death. Attendees received a flyer and, if interested, signed up for one of six focus groups to be outside the conference schedule. A maximum of 12 attendees could sign up for a given group. Group sizes ranged from one to ten participants (mean = 6, SD = 4).

The focus groups lasted about one hour. Two RAND project staff members were present during each session: One led the group and the other took detailed notes on a laptop computer. All focus groups were audiorecorded and followed a written protocol of open-ended questions. Each session had three goals: (1) to elicit perspectives on the issues and needs of military suicide loss survivors, (2) to gauge how loss survivors felt DoD was doing in addressing their needs, and (3) to strategize how DoD might better meet loss survivors' needs following a suicide. Participants gave verbal consent to participate and received food and refreshments for their participation. As part of the camp protocol, licensed mental health professionals were available outside each meeting room in case any clinical issues arose. No referrals to these professionals were necessary during any of the group sessions.

Qualitative Data Analyses

After the focus groups, two RAND research team members independently reviewed the audiotapes, transcripts, and notes. The purpose of this review was to identify, label, and group key points that spoke to loss survivors' recommendations. Using grounded theory analysis (see Strauss, 1998), we grouped key points with similar themes into a category if they were mentioned several times (e.g., CAOs provided support; see Ryan and Bernard, 2003). We then discussed each of the categories and generated underlying themes from the data (e.g., experiences with CAOs or CACOs have been varied and effective). After we extracted these themes, we used classic content analysis to identify quotes that fit each theme (Krippendorff, 2004; Weber, 1990). Each researcher independently sorted quotes by theme and then, together, reached a consensus where there were discrepancies.

Sample

A total of 34 (29 female and five male) military loss survivors aged 18 years and older participated in one of six focus groups (see Table 6.1). Of the 34 participants, 19 were immediate family members (15 parents, three siblings, one aunt), and 15 were spouses. The length of time since the suicide varied. About 32 percent of the sample had lost their loved one within the prior year, 38 percent two to three years ago, and 26 percent four or more years ago. One participant did not disclose how long ago the death had occurred.

Results

Table 6.2 summarizes identified themes and related quotes from the loss survivor focus groups. In general, survivors commented on their personal experiences and focused their recommendations on how the military could help future military loss survivors.

Varied Experiences with Casualty Assistance Officers

Participants reported varied experiences with CAOs or CACOs but found them effective. This was the most common theme among all the groups and was often the first issue raised in each discussion. Several participants said that they were paired with an officer who was caring, helpful, and knowledgeable, while other participants were paired with an officer who presumably lacked empathy and knowledge about the grief process and the military administrative process.

Table 6.1
Loss Survivor Focus Group Demographics

Characteristic	Number
Gender	
Female	29
Male	5
Relationship to decedent	
Parent	15
Sibling	3
Aunt	1
Spouse	15
Time since death (years)	
< 1	4
1	7
2–3	13
4–5	6
> 5	3
Total	34

Table 6.2
Themes from TAPS Focus Groups with Suicide Loss Survivors

Theme	Quotes from Loss Survivors
Experiences with CAOs or CACOs have been varied and effective.	"The CAO is a really important part of the process for us."
	"The CACOs need a resource for them. I had too many times where I had to go out and find answers for myself."
Administrative documents and processes are overwhelming and challenging to navigate.	"It took me three years to be able to understand some of the paperwork. [At first I was] just filling out forms. I'm still a little hazy."
	"[You need] paperwork filled out, and to have things explained more."
Grief resources and support services are challenging to navigate.	"Leave no man on the field. Some families are left alone, which is just like leaving a man on the field."
	"My handbook [of information and resources] was this big [holding hands wide]."
	"I didn't hear about TAPS until three years [after the death]. There are other groups in the civilian world that are able to help, including Compassionate Friends, [Survivor Outreach Services], and the United Way. Some kind of list for civilians [would help]."
Suicide deaths are treated differently.	"You're treated differently."
	"The focus shouldn't be the manner of death. . . . It should be that they served."
Parents/next of kin are treated differently from spouses.	"The family is the family. Don't just provide services to the next of kin or spouse. Parents are treated like garbage."
	"Need the same level of services for the parents and other kin as for the spouses."
	"Even in good situations, the spouse or sibling has different needs."

Participants had different experiences with their officers, but it was clear that being paired with an officer who was both warm and knowledgeable made a significant difference in their experience. One loss survivor articulated this point, stating that the CAO "was dressed in uniform and when I tried to give him a handshake he gave me a hug. This showed me that the military cared. He did that with my children as well. He connected with us right away. He was following military protocol, straight and narrow, but was warm." Another participant said, "I had a great CACO! He initiated everything. Whatever questions I had, he made appointments. He walked me through all the steps and made appointments with retirement specialists and also attended these meetings." In contrast, another spouse commented that it felt like the CAO was "inconvenienced" each time they visited, and another spouse felt the CAO was not knowledgeable or helpful with administrative processes.

Many participants who reflected on their CAO experience speculated that this variation might be due to a lack of standardized training for the officers. One loss survivor noted that the training is different at each location: "It's just so unequal." Participants recommended more standardized training in grief support and administrative paperwork to help CAOs compassionately support loss survivors and assist them with navigating administrative processes (e.g., what benefits are available).

Overwhelming Administrative Documents and Processes

The second theme that emerged was that loss survivors perceived administrative documents and processes, which they are encouraged to complete soon after the death, as overwhelming and challenging to navigate. Administrative documents and processes included funeral arrangements, insurance, trust funds, belongings, life insurance, the cause-of-death investigation, and Servicemembers Group Life Insurance benefits. Loss survivors commented that administrative paperwork was confusing and required multiple calls to different agencies. They said they felt pressured because important decisions needed to be made in a timely manner. In the words of to one loss survivor, "For me, dealing with the benefits . . . it was just confusing." According to another, "There are legal documents that need to be signed, and you're not sure whether you should or shouldn't sign [them]." Loss survivors repeatedly recommended that they be provided with someone to walk them through the various administrative documents and processes.

Loss survivors also noted that the process of investigating the details of the event was difficult to understand. They found it difficult to get information about what happened to the decedent. "When you start asking questions . . . that's when the walls go up," said one loss survivor. Another said of the investigative process, "[The] time was long, [and] the process wasn't clear. [It] needed to be transparent." Loss survivors stated that the time required for the investigation was emotionally challenging because they would reexperience the news of their loved one's death each time updates were available.

The "Fog" After the Loss

Many loss survivors talked about being "in a fog" after their loss, which revealed a third theme. Loss survivors stated that grief resources and support services were challenging to navigate and too overwhelming to sort through. They reported receiving a "handbook" of resources that was unclear and too extensive to review right after the suicide. One asked, "Who has time to read a book?" Another said, "It's such a shock [and] you're at such a loss." "You don't know what you need," added another. Many loss survivors also reported not hearing about TAPS and other support services right away, and sometimes not until years after the death, and said they had to find these resources on their own. Some participants commented that it would be helpful to have a designated person who proactively called and provided resources. Some participants felt that it was difficult to reach out for help but that they would have accepted it if offered. For example, one participant said, "If you don't 'take the stigma out,' people don't get the help when they need it." Recommendations to address these issues included having one broad fact sheet accompanied by specific brochures on various resources. In addition, some loss survivors suggested that the CAO should help navigate the numerous resources and services, stating that "[a] trained CACO that gives the person as much information as they need [is important]."

Differing Treatment of Suicide Deaths and Other Deaths

Another theme that emerged was that suicide deaths were treated differently from deaths by other means. Most participants felt resentment that their loved ones had served their country but were treated differently from other service members who had not died by suicide. One loss survivor said that suicide decedents were not given the same "honor or glory." Loss survivors said that various recognitions were not provided. For example, there was no gun salute at the funeral or motorcade, and the President did not send a letter to the family when the death was from suicide. In addition, families were not considered "gold star" if the service member died by suicide. Loss survivors also noted that there were two tiers of pins given to families: one for families of service members who were killed in action and a lower tier of pins for suicide loss survivors. One loss survivor said, "Give everybody the honor." Overall, loss survivors recommended that those who die by suicide and their survivors receive the same recognition and benefits that are afforded to other service members and their families.

Differing Treatment of Family Members and Spouses

Finally, loss survivors felt that parents or next of kin of the suicide decedent were treated differently from their spouses and that more services were needed for other family members who required the same amount of support. One loss survivor said, "The CACO did explain the benefits—[my son] was married so I wasn't the primary survivor, [and his wife] may have received more information than I did—but there should be something where the parents should get the same type of information [as others]." In some cases, the parents or next of kin and spouses received different information from the military. For example, one loss survivor stated, "Each of us had our own CAO, and the CAOs were relaying messages. I didn't think about the funeral until a few days after hearing about the death, and the CAO told me, 'Don't worry about it.' Later, I found out that my mother-in-law was [planning the funeral]." Other loss survivors agreed: "Everyone needs to see the same information so there's no room for interpretation," "Don't just talk with spouse," and "Take into consideration the total family!" Assigning the parents and spouses the same CAOs was frequently recommended to improve the communication of important information to both types of loss survivors.

Conclusion

The goals of this portion of the study were to evaluate the experiences of military suicide loss survivors after the death of a loved one. Loss survivors described varying experiences with their CAOs but generally found these officers effective. They also found administrative documents and processes to be challenging, had difficulty navigating available grief and support resources, believed that suicide deaths were treated differently from other military deaths, and thought that parents and next of kin were treated differently from spouses. In the aftermath of their loved one's death, loss survivors expressed a range of experiences, and the quality of their interactions with various military processes seemed to affect how were adjusting emotionally.

The study results presented here provide a focused examination of military loss survivors and the involvement of parents, siblings, and spouses across military branches and geographical areas. However, these results are not necessarily generalizable to all military suicide loss survivors. Our focus groups were held at one military loss survivor camp and thus represent only the focus group participants who volunteered for the study. It is unknown how loss survivors who did not want to participate or who did not attend the camp felt. Future studies could examine loss survivors' views across other camps or in other settings that reach loss survivor populations to capture the full spectrum of loss survivor experiences.

Even though the findings are not generalizable, they still have several important implications. First, the military has a significant opportunity to help facilitate the bereavement of loss survivors through the careful selection and training of CAOs, by streamlining administrative processes and documents, and by facilitating referrals. Second, loss survivors also have a tremendous opportunity to help each other by requesting the reassignment of CAOs when there is a poor match and by helping to inform fellow loss survivors of resources they may take advantage of. As seen through our focus groups, multiple factors likely affect loss survivors, including their social support system, coping strategies, and the military's response to their loved one's death.

Two themes of inequity were raised. First, loss survivors felt that suicide deaths were treated differently from other types of deaths. Several recent policy changes have been made that may not have been captured in the participating loss survivors' comments. For example, in July 2011, President Obama adjusted the policy for condolence letters, which previously had not been sent to service members who committed suicide in a combat zone. In his statement, he acknowledged the importance of honoring service to the nation and removing the stigma surrounding suicide (White House, 2011). In addition, the military now has policies and procedures that describe memorial and funeral offerings available to deceased military personnel, as well as awards and honors that they are eligible to receive posthumously. These changes have changed the manner in which the military treats suicide deaths. Considerable stigma may still surround suicide deaths. Thus, how loss survivors perceive and grieve their loved one's death is often influenced by how other groups, including the military and society, perceive suicide.

The second theme of inequity involved how parents felt they were treated compared with spouses. Parents, overall, felt that spouses received more information and resources. While we did not collect marital and demographic information on the decedents, this perspective may be related to the young age at which most service members enlist. For example, parents may want a more active role in cases in which their child was married for only a short time. Future research is needed to examine the impact of suicide on young families. Parents were understandably affected by their child's death and felt that more attention to them would have helped their bereavement.

While efforts to prevent suicide among members of the armed forces continue, the military has always experienced and will in the foreseeable future continue to experience suicide among its ranks. Thus, efforts to understand how to facilitate the bereavement process for loss survivors are both important and meaningful. As seen from our results, the military has an influence on how family members grieve, and their experiences are significantly variable. The military is a unique culture, and caring for its loss survivors is necessary to honor and pay respect to loss survivors and their loved ones.

CHAPTER SEVEN

Recommendations

The objectives of this study were to identify the policies and procedures in place in DoD and across the services for responding to suicide and to document the extent to which DoD programs and policies reflect state-of-the-art suicide postvention practices. Unfortunately, the evidence is so sparse in this area that it is challenging to identify the state of the art. The gold standard of scientific evidence—randomized control trials—is practically nonexistent in this area, and the bulk of the evidence derives from expert opinion. Given this shortcoming, it is surprising that we identified more than 600 unique recommendations from available published guides, which we tried to catalogue in a systematic way, describing the level of evidence available for each grouping.

Nonetheless, in the process of conducting this research, we were able to develop 11 recommendations rooted in some level of evidence or consensus. These recommendations span the following seven areas:

1. Further strengthen the existing military suicide surveillance system by adding data elements to the DoDSER, enumerating suicide rates among members of the reserve component, and conducting in-depth investigations on suicide decedents.
2. Prepare an organizational response to suicide by developing a plan that specifies actions and responsible actors and ensures sufficient resources.
3. Work with the media to encourage factual reporting and minimize sensationalism of suicides.
4. Identify individuals at high risk.
5. Establish greater uniformity across CAOs in the ways they handle suicide deaths, consistent with standards.
6. Educate leaders, CAOs, and other support personnel about complicated grief; train health care providers on evidence-based treatments.
7. Reconsider whether eligibility for DoD and VA benefits should be affected by LoD determinations, and support loss survivors in making informed decisions about benefits.

Strengthen the Existing Suicide Surveillance System

The first three recommendations pertain to strengthening the existing suicide surveillance system by adding elements to the DoDSER, enumerating suicide rates among members of the reserve component, and conducting in-depth investigations on suicide decedents. DoD's suicide surveillance program generally surpasses those in the civilian sector, particularly for active-duty service members. Nonetheless, we provide three recommendations here that could strengthen an already strong system.

Recommendation 1. Incorporate fields into the DoDSER that identify data sources and the timing and severity thresholds for stressful life events.
To the extent possible, it is critical that surveillance elements be standardized. Reflecting the CDC's recommendations on core data elements, including the source for each data element would help ensure that information is being categorized consistently. In addition, according to best practices for conducting psychological autopsies, identifying the thresholds and timing of stressful life events would enhance standardization. This level of detail does exist for some fields (i.e., deployment history), but efforts should be made to ensure that all life stressors have a similar level of detail.

Recommendation 2. Create a process to enumerate suicides among reservists and members of the National Guard not on active duty.
Suicide surveillance among military personnel is primarily focused on members of the active component and reservists and members of the National Guard on active duty. There is currently no systematic process for conducting surveillance for members of the National Guard or reserves who are not on active duty. Existing strategies are ad hoc, and it is not clear whether DoD procedures capture all suicide deaths among this group. Linking DoD and National Death Index data, as advocated by others (e.g., Miller et al., 2012), would be a first step in an effort to conduct comprehensive suicide surveillance for this population.

Recommendation 3. Conduct psychological autopsies on all or a sample of confirmed suicides and on a specified control group on an ongoing basis.
Information gleaned from the DoDSER could be enhanced on an ongoing basis with information from psychological autopsies conducted on all or a sample of military suicides and on a specified control group. Such a system can help identify the degree to which an antecedent confers suicide risk. For example, if the proportion of service members who filed for divorce is higher among suicide decedents in the three months prior to death than among a matched control group, that may indicate that the three months following a divorce filing is a risk period for possible suicide. Thus, the surveillance strategy can help inform a strategy for implementing targeted suicide prevention programs. However, it is imperative that such investigations be conducted in a systematic way that minimizes bias. Thus, interviewers should be recruited and trained specifically for this purpose, and the protocols and procedures they follow should be consistent.

Establish an Organizational Response to Suicide

Our second category of recommendations pertains to preparing a plan that specifies actions and responsible actors and ensures that sufficient resources are in place to mount an appropriate organizational response to suicide. While certain DoD suborganizations and installations may have plans for responding to suicides, there does not appear to be a significant degree of uniformity in these responses. There also does not appear to be an overarching DoD-wide or service-wide plan or a directive for suborganizations or installations to develop such a plan. Suicides bring a great deal of emotional upheaval and confusion, and it is important for responses to be swift to be effective. Therefore, plans for how to respond should already be in place and easy to implement. We provide two recommendations specific to preparing a plan to respond.

Recommendation 4: Ensure that installations and military organizations are ready to respond to suicide with a detailed plan, dedicated staff responsible for implementing the plan, and sufficient resources to enact the plan.

The CDC guidelines listed in Chapter Three should be followed to the extent possible and referenced when drafting a plan. Given the size of the military and variation across installations, a "one-size-fits-all" plan may not be feasible. Thus, DoD might consider whether different plans are needed for different contexts (e.g., for personnel on deployment) or for the different services. The plan should include the specific actions that will be taken and who will be responsible for each.

Suborganizations and installations should ensure that leaders are aware of the plan before a suicide occurs, and they should be responsible and accountable for carrying it out when a suicide does occur. The leadership should nominate a team of individuals who know plan components and are responsible for ensuring that it gets enacted. This team may include members both within the organization and in the community who may be called upon to assist after a suicide; at the very least, one or more members of the team should have preestablished relationships with these outside organizations and communicate with them about the suicide and how the organization is planning to respond. Training leaders and those responsible for enacting the plan prior to a suicide will help ensure that parties responsible for carrying out the prescribed details are aware of their responsibilities and can perform them effectively.

Recommendation 5: Ensure that installations include in their suicide response plan a process for guiding any memorial services they conduct.

There is no scientific evidence regarding the benefits of memorials or how they should be conducted. However, the existing data suggest some ways to determine how best to memorialize those who die by suicide. The military has its own community and culture that influence attitudes about suicide (and may differ among the services), but decedents and bereaved loss survivors' cultures and communities of origin might have attitudes about death and suicide that conflict with the military's. It is important to be aware of the decedent's and his or her family's cultural and religious background and to take this into consideration in planning memorials.

There need not necessarily be a prescribed plan that treats all suicides the same way. Instead a response plan would benefit from a standardized process for determining whether to hold a memorial service and the content of that service. This determination may be made by a consensus of key organizational or installation representatives (e.g., installation leader, chaplain, unit leader), but it should also include representation from the decedent's family. In addition, physical memorials (e.g., plaques, statues, tree plantings) should be considered cautiously.

Work with the Media to Encourage Factual Reporting and Minimize Sensationalism of Suicides

The inappropriate presentation of suicides in the media can be harmful and promote contagion. There is some evidence that effective dissemination of media guidelines can improve the quality of reporting (Pirkis, Dare, et al., 2009), but it may be equally important for individual organizations to work collaboratively with the media to avoid potentially harmful coverage.

Recommendation 6: View the media as a partner and encourage journalists to comply with the media guidelines.
Military suicides are often high-profile and of great interest to the media, so media reporting has the potential to prevent or promote future suicides. Table 3.2 presents guidelines for the media on how to respond to suicides. Military press outlets should be aware of these guidelines, and the personnel responsible for interacting with the media—preferably specified in the plan described in recommendation 3—should encourage their external media partners to abide by them.

Identify Individuals at High Risk

A suicide may heighten the risk of suicide for already vulnerable individuals. Identifying those who are at an increased risk for suicide is one of six components of a comprehensive response to suicide and should be a specific consideration after a suicide.

Recommendation 7: Implement a systematic process for identifying and referring at-risk individuals.
There is some evidence from studies in schools that widespread mental health and suicide screening may help identify individuals in need of mental health treatment, but it is not clear whether such findings are reliable or generalizable to the military. Therefore, we cannot make recommendations for or against broad or universal screening after a suicide at this time. However, systematic screening after a suicide of subpopulations *known* to be at elevated risk for suicide (e.g., due to previously identified depression, a history of suicide attempts, or being a close friend or family member of the decedent) could facilitate referral to or enhancement of treatment, thus lowering suicide risk. For example, after a suicide, behavioral health providers could reassess their patients for suicidal ideation and intent and alter their treatment plans accordingly. While encouraging and training supervisors and peers to pay close attention to suicide loss survivors may be common, the evidence to date does not suggest that these more informal processes can identify all of those who are most at risk. Furthermore, such a strategy should not isolate or stigmatize those who are identified.

Individuals trained as gatekeepers (e.g., chaplains, noncommissioned officers), as well as CAOs, are also likely to be exposed to populations at the highest risk (e.g., loss survivors experiencing intense grief and hopelessness) following a suicide and may be well positioned to implement new screening procedures. However, this will require additional support and resources, including increased time for screening and referral, to perform such tasks effectively.

Because of the overall lack of research on screening, particularly after a suicide, well-controlled studies to test screening protocols are needed and should be planned in advance. For example, after a suicide, a screening procedure could be implemented and possibly randomly assigned to similar test and control groups. Group differences in the identification of individuals previously not known to be at risk, or referral to or participation in treatment or support groups, could be measured outcomes.

Establish Greater Uniformity Across CAOs in How They Handle Suicide Deaths, Consistent with Standards

CAOs play a critical role after a suicide, from notifying family members of a death to helping them negotiate administrative responsibilities. However, even the small group of loss survivors we spoke with had very different experiences with their CAOs.

Recommendation 8: Prioritize reducing variability in the quality of CAOs.
This may require imposing stricter requirements for CAOs and potentially making only certain career fields eligible to serve in this role. CAOs should be sensitive to the unique needs of those who experience a loss. However, they should not treat suicide loss survivors differently with respect to informing them and making them aware of the rights and honors that are available to the decedent and the family.

Educate Leaders, CAOs, and Other Support Personnel About the Grieving Process, Including Complicated Grief, and Train Providers in Evidence-Based Treatments

Loss survivors may grieve in different ways and need different levels and types of support. While the majority go through the grieving process without experiencing clinically significant symptoms, it is estimated that between 7 and 25 percent of bereaved individuals experience complicated grief. They may be family members of the deceased but also friends, colleagues, and unit members. Leaders, CAOs, and behavioral health professionals should be made aware of typical and complicated grief so that they can encourage access to evidence-based care by those who may benefit from support or treatment.

Recommendation 9: Make leaders and CAOs aware that grief is a normal process following death, and sudden deaths may produce different and unique manifestations of grief.
Individuals have unique ways to cope with their grief: Some may seek support from family or friends, and others may seek support from religious personnel or choose to grieve alone. Leaders and CAOs should ensure that loss survivors have access to the many and varied resources available to them. They should also be alert to and discourage maladaptive coping behaviors (e.g., excessive alcohol use). In addition, the amount of time it takes an individual to grieve may vary; some loss survivors might need ongoing monitoring and support. "Checking-in" on loss survivors to ensure that they are learning to adapt to their new life situation is critical. Those who are not adapting may be developing complicated grief and should be encouraged to seek the services of a behavioral health professional who can provide evidence-based care.

Recommendation 10: Ensure that care providers and others (e.g., military psychologists and psychiatrists, mental health providers, family counselors) who may come into contact with grieving loss survivors are aware of the symptoms of complicated grief and trained in effective cognitive behavioral approaches.
While there is no evidence that complicated grief can be prevented, there is evidence that those suffering from complicated grief can improve when offered certain types of treatments, such as cognitive behavioral therapy. For a summary of the evidence regarding the efficacy of treatments for complicated grief, see Table 4.1 in Chapter Four.

Reconsider Whether Eligibility for DoD and VA Benefits Should Be Affected by LoD Determinations, and Support Loss Survivors in Making Informed Decisions About Benefits

Those who lose someone to suicide should not be punished for the way in which their loved one died. Thus, equality should be ensured for those entitled to benefits. When dispensing benefits, DoD should be sensitive to the administrative burdens associated with accessing these benefits, particularly among those who have suffered a sudden loss.

Recommendation 11. Consider modifying eligibility for loss survivor benefits and dependency and indemnity compensation to ensure that suicide loss survivors have access to these benefits.
Instrumental to ensuring equality is to ensure that family members of suicide decedents have access to the same benefits as the family members of service members who die by other means. Currently, access to DoD's Survivor Benefit Plan and the VA's Dependency and Indemnity Compensation may be denied to suicide loss survivors due to the results of the LoD investigation.

There is reasonable concern that the provision of benefits to suicide loss survivors may act as an incentive for those at risk to choose to take their lives. This is an important point and why we recommend that DoD *consider* modifying eligibility, perhaps only after studying this issue more closely. However, this hypothesis needs to be balanced by policies that already extend benefits to suicide loss survivors. If the provision of benefits does act as an incentive, should loss survivors be eligible for *any* benefits? If not, why should some benefits be denied for suicide deaths determined not in the line of duty?

Recommendation 12: Ensure that the timing and presentation of benefits take into account loss survivors' ability to process this information in the acute period following their loss.
Many loss survivors we spoke with described being in a "fog" when told about or discovering their loved one's suicide. DoD should recognize that this may impede their ability to make important decisions and sort through piles of information independently. CAOs should offer to help suicide loss survivors process this information, not only in the immediate aftermath of a death but also on an ongoing basis as survivors come to terms with their loss.

Conclusion

This report is intended to help military leaders respond to suicide in a way that reflects improved understanding of suicide within the ranks and that supports its members, including families, who are dealing with a sudden and tragic loss. Rather than add to the myriad resource guides that already exist, this report provides a scientific foundation for understanding the recommendations that have been made to help organizations respond to suicide, and it compiles these recommendations in a single source. By following the 12 recommendations presented here, which in many cases align with recommendations made elsewhere, DoD can respond to suicides in a respectful way—and in a way that may help prevent future suicides.

APPENDIX A

Postvention Guides Reviewed

Table A.1 lists the postvention guides reviewed for this study. The table presents citation information and notes the format of the guide (e.g., journal article, video, checklist). Some of the guides are available online; URLs for those resources can be found in the bibliography.

Table A.1
Postvention Guides Reviewed

Title	Creator	Publisher	Date	Format
"After a Suicide" (crisis response planning for schools)	Youth Suicide Prevention Program	Youth Suicide Prevention Program	2003	Fact sheet
"After a Suicide: A Postvention Primer for Providers," *MCES Quest*, Vol. 5, No. 2, December 2006	Montgomery County (Pa.) Emergency Medical Services, Inc.	Montgomery County (Pa.) Emergency Medical Services, Inc.	2006	Newsletter
After a Suicide: Recommendations for Religious Services and Other Public Memorial Observances	Suicide Prevention Resource Center	Education Development Center, Inc.	2004	Report
"CDC Recommendations for a Community Plan for the Prevention and Containment of Suicide Clusters," *Morbidity and Mortality Weekly*, Vol. 37, Suppl. 6	Centers for Disease Control and Prevention	Centers for Disease Control and Prevention	1988	Article
Coming Together to Care: A Suicide Prevention and Postvention Toolkit for Texas Communities	Texas Suicide Prevention Community Network	Mental Health America of Texas	2009	Toolkit
Community-Based Suicide Prevention Guidelines for Wisconsin	Mental Health America of Wisconsin	Mental Health America of Wisconsin	2010	Toolkit
Coping After a Suicide	Families for Depression Awareness	Families for Depression Awareness	2008	Brochure
Crisis Intervention: A Guide for School-Based Clinicians	Center for School Mental Health Assistance	University of Maryland	2002	Study guide
"Culturally Competent Crisis Response: Information for School Psychologists and Crisis Teams"	National Association of School Psychologists	National Association of School Psychologists	2004	Fact sheet
"Dealing with Death at School," *Principal Leadership Magazine*	Poland, Scott, and Donna Poland	National Association of School Psychologists	2004	Article
"For Parents"	Society for the Prevention of Teen Suicide	Society for the Prevention of Teen Suicide	Undated	Website
"For Professionals: Considerations for School Settings"	Centre for Suicide Prevention (Canada)	Centre for Suicide Prevention (Canada)	2005	Checklist
Garrett Lee Smith Youth Suicide Prevention Toolkit	Mental Health America of Wisconsin	Mental Health America of Wisconsin	2007	Information package

Table A.1—Continued

Title	Creator	Publisher	Date	Format
"Helping Students Cope with Suicide"	Evans, Robert	National Association of Independent Schools	2004	Fact sheet
"How Can Emergency Responders Help Grieving Individuals?"	Lerner, Mark D., and Raymond D. Shelton	American Academy of Experts in Traumatic Stress	2001	Article
"In the Wake of Trauma: Tips for College Students"	Substance Abuse and Mental Health Services Administration	Substance Abuse and Mental Health Services Administration	2010	Information package
Lifeline Online Suicide Prevention Manual	National Suicide Prevention Lifeline	Substance Abuse and Mental Health Services Administration	2010	Information package
"Managing School Crises: More Than Just Response," *Principal Leadership Magazine*	Reeves, Melissa A., Stephen E. Brock, Katherine C. Cowan	National Association of Secondary School Principals	2008	Article
"Media Guidelines for School Administrators Who May Interact with Reporters About Youth Suicide"	Maine Youth Suicide Prevention Program	Maine Department of Health and Human Services	2007	Policy guidelines
"Memorial Activities at School: A List of 'Dos' and 'Don'ts'"	National Association of School Psychologists	National Association of School Psychologists	2002	Fact sheet
"The Police and Mental Health," *Psychiatry Online*, Vol. 53, No. 10	Lamb, H. Richard, Linda E. Weinberger, and Walter J. DeCuir, Jr.	*Psychiatry Online*	2002	Article
Postvention Standards Manual: A Guide for a School's Response in the Aftermath of Sudden Death, 4th ed.	Kerr, Mary Margaret, David A. Brent, Brian McKain, and Paula S. McCommons	STAR Center, Division of Child Psychiatry, University of Pittsburgh Medical Center	2010	Manual
Preventing Suicide: How to Start a Survivors' Group	World Health Organization and International Association for Suicide Prevention	World Health Organization Press	2008	Monograph
Reporting on Suicide: Recommendations for the Media	Centers for Disease Control and Prevention, National Institute of Mental Health, Office of the Surgeon General, Substance Abuse and Mental Health Services Administration, American Foundation for Suicide Prevention, American Association of Suicidology, and Annenberg Public Policy Center	American Foundation for Suicide Prevention	2001	Information package

Table A.1—Continued

Title	Creator	Publisher	Date	Format
School-Based Crisis Management: Recommendations on Suicide	Suicide Awareness Voices of Education	Suicide Awareness Voices of Education	2007	Policy guidelines
School-Based Suicide Prevention: A Matter of Life and Death	Ulrich, Jan	Kentucky Cabinet for Health and Family Services	2009	Video
"School Memorials After Suicide: Helpful or Harmful?" *SEIC Alert*, No. 54	Centre for Suicide Prevention (Canada)	Centre for Suicide Prevention (Canada)	2004	Fact sheet
Supporting Survivors of Suicide Loss: A Guide for Funeral Directors	Suicide Prevention Action Network USA and Suicide Prevention Resource Center	Suicide Prevention Action Network USA and Suicide Prevention Resource Center	2008	Brochure

APPENDIX B

Content Analysis of Resource Guides

This appendix presents each unique recommendation identified in the 41 documents listed in Appendix A, along with the categories into which we collapsed the recommendations (step 2 of the process described in Chapter One, labeled A, B, C, and so on) and the 31 broad categories into which we collapsed the recommendation categories as described in step 3 in Chapter One (labeled 1, 2, 3, and so on). For more details about these methods, see the section "Analysis of Resource Guides" in Chapter One. This appendix concludes with a list of recommendations that were excluded from the analysis and our justification for excluding them.

1. *Care for care providers.* Those who provide emotional or spiritual support may also be grieving the loss and may, at times, find it difficult to provide care. They should be reminded and encouraged to take care of their own individual well-being.
   A. *Monitor and care for care providers.*
      - Provide postvention care to care providers who may have treated patients who have died by suicide.
      - Monitor the mental health of care providers and treatment staff.

   B. *Remind care providers (psychiatrists, psychologists, social workers, chaplains) to take care of their own, personal needs.*
      - Adopt the same approach as used for loss survivors to deal with grief.
      - Be gentle with yourself and others.
      - Be kind and patient with yourself.
      - Be mindful of effects of crisis on adults in a school.
      - "Be with your grief."
      - Consider being with friends.
      - Do not hesitate to seek counseling.
      - Engage in self-monitoring.
      - Get support for your own feelings.
      - Ignore negative words from others.
      - Monitor personal processing and support needs.
      - Seek professional help if necessary.
      - Take care of yourself.
      - Use relaxation, meditation, or prayer.
      - Deal with your own reactions first.
      - Leaders or care providers must pay attention to their own needs.

2. *Promote collaboration among organizations.* Those responding to suicide should work collaboratively with internal stakeholders and external agencies (e.g., the media, law enforcement, local support agencies). Relationships may be formal or informal and, when possible, established prior to a suicide event.
   A. *People and organizations should work collaboratively to support loss survivors.*
      ◦ Work collaboratively to support the loss survivor.
   B. *Collaborate with community entities (e.g., media, law enforcement, local support agencies.*
      ◦ Collaborate with the media, law enforcement, and community agencies.
      ◦ Develop a system for contacting necessary crisis resources.
      ◦ Contact the local mental health agency.
      ◦ Contact the police when necessary.
      ◦ Notify community resources and discuss collaboration.
      ◦ Police departments should participate in specialized mobile crisis response teams.
   C. *Coordinate with community providers and other resources.*
      ◦ Coordinate with local schools and community providers.
      ◦ Engage the community, including communication with other schools and groups.
      ◦ Reach out to other schools in district.
      ◦ Teams should preestablish strong relationships with important resources and figures in community.
      ◦ Coordinate a response with the community.
      ◦ Coordinate with community organizations and all relevant institutional bodies.
      ◦ Coordinate with local mental health or crisis response resources.
      ◦ Develop memorandums of agreement with local crisis agencies.
      ◦ Develop school-community partnerships.
      ◦ Engage support from other designated school personnel.
      ◦ Contact the school counselor, nurse, and 911.
      ◦ Network with community institutions.
      ◦ Police and mental health departments should collaborate closely.
      ◦ A response should also include community resources able to help, such as clergy and the police.
      ◦ A response should involve all necessary agencies with one leading plan.
      ◦ Groups should engage in coalition-building to lessen the burden.
      ◦ Collaborate with regional, local, and school leaders, among others.

3. *Ensure confidentiality.* Confidentiality protocols should be prepared in advance to protect loss survivors' privacy.
   A. *Do not to rely on loss survivors' family or friends, due to privacy/confidentiality issues.*
      ◦ Do not use loss survivors' friends or relatives for community outreach or translation or interpretation, due to confidentiality issues.
   B. *Establish a confidentiality protocol.*
      ◦ Discuss and establish a confidentiality protocol.
   C. *Maintain privacy when aiding and assisting loss survivors.*
      ◦ Respect loss survivors' privacy. Share information with staff only when necessary.

4. *Create groups, places, and spaces.* Resources available for loss survivors' public expressions of grief should include support groups and physical spaces.
   A. *Develop and run a self-help group.*
      - Develop and run a self-help group.
   B. *Establish a place to grieve and provide permission for loss survivors to grieve.*
      - Provide permission to grieve and a place to grieve.
      - Designate a crisis center area.
      - Establish a support center.

5. *Promote cultural sensitivity.* Responders should recognize and accommodate the cultural context of the loss survivor community.
   A. *Postvention messages should be culturally sensitive.*
      - Help loss survivors find comfort within the context of their faith or faith community.
      - Be attentive to cultural considerations among minority populations.
      - Be aware of other environmental challenges in loss survivors' lives.
      - Consider the special needs of youth.
      - Recruit assistance from minority populations during crisis response planning.
      - Respect loss survivors' faith and spirituality.
      - Understand that loss survivors react within the context of their individual backgrounds.
      - Use age-appropriate therapy to help children adjust after a traumatic event.
      - Be sensitive to developmental and cultural differences.
      - Dress appropriately for the local cultural context.
      - Ensure that responses reflect cultural and religious differences.
      - Use interpreters to provide culturally appropriate messages.
      - Use the language of the population or interpreters.
      - Be aware of cultural differences in styles of communication, body language, etc.
      - Disseminate timely information to community in languages other than English.
      - Use the correct courtesy gestures and greetings.
      - Take special language and cultural considerations into account.
      - Make sure form letters are available in multiple languages.
      - Organize culturally appropriate memorials or other commemoration activities.
      - Use teams to assess the effectiveness and cultural competence of interventions.
      - Cultural competency should include an interpreter, if necessary, and an understanding of relevant cultural norms regarding death, pain, and suffering.
      - Make use of cross-cultural interventions.
      - Acknowledge cultural limitations and differences.
      - Increase one's own awareness of cultural issues.
      - Maintain a profile of the cultural or demographic composition of institution or community (e.g., socioeconomic status, age, gender, religion, rural versus urban, communal experiences of subpopulations).
      - Recognize the cultural effects on traumatic reactions.
      - Refer loss survivors to culturally appropriate resources.
      - Assemble a crisis team that reflects the cultural or demographic makeup of the client population.

- Involve individuals and subgroups from diverse backgrounds in the response plan.
- Keep a list of the full names of parents and guardians, as naming traditions can vary.
- Conduct a crisis response evaluation that includes cultural considerations.
- Be aware of taboos, including those involving gender, socioeconomic status, ethnic background, etc.
- Crisis response should be tailored to the population in need.
- Include crisis responders and culture brokers from minority groups at all phases of the response.
- Identify potential translators or interpreters.
- Prepare form letters in advance in multiple languages.
- Identify the specific needs of the community.
- Understand the cultural context of the event.
- Understand the demographics of the school.
- Tailor support services for students with special needs.

B. *Be deliberately inclusive.*
- Reach out and draw loss survivors into the community.
- Provide permission to grieve and a place to grieve.
- Practice deliberate inclusiveness.
- Designate a crisis center area.

6. *Ensure proper documentation.* Documentation following a suicide should include verification of the cause of death by external authorities. Other documents should track internal actions and loss survivor contact information.

A. *Confirm the cause of death with appropriate officials (e.g., medical examiner, police).*
- Confirm the death with appropriate officials.
- Develop and run a self-help group.
- Contact law enforcement to verify the facts of the case.
- Verify that the cause of death was suicide.
- Verify that the cause of death has been determined.
- Verify the death.

B. *Document the actions taken and decisions made after a suicide.*
- Report on activities coordinated by the local or state suicide-prevention coalition.
- Provide permission to grieve and a place to grieve.
- Document actions taken.
- Designate a crisis center area.
- Document all information pertaining to the student's attempt, the school's follow-up, and the parents' response.
- Establish a support center.
- Keep an informal procedures log.
- Keep records of training for legal liability.

C. *Develop a roster of decedents' family members.*
- Identify full names of parents and guardians of schoolchildren.
- Inform the school superintendent and administrators about siblings.

7. *Conduct an environmental risk assessment.* Environmental elements that might increase the risk of suicide contagion should be identified and addressed.
   A. *Identify and address environmental elements that might increase fatal suicides.*
      - Focus on the building and people during recovery.
      - Confirm the death with the appropriate officials.
      - Develop and run a self-help group.
      - Know the community and surrounding hazards.
      - Contact law enforcement to verify the facts of the case.
      - Know the school building and assess potential hazards.
      - Verify that the cause of death was suicide.
      - Identify and address environmental elements that might increase suicide risk.
      - Verify that the cause of death has been determined.
      - Address environmental elements that might increase the likelihood of further suicides.
      - Verify the death.

8. *Foster a supportive community.* Community development efforts should include direct discussion about suicide misconceptions and support services should encourage positive connections among service members, leaders, and support personnel.
   A. *Attack stigma.*
      - Attack stigma: Disclose selected information about the context, discuss factors commonly associated with suicide, and dispel myths about moral weakness character flaws.
      - Contact law enforcement to verify the facts of the case.
      - Be realistic about the services that can be provided.
      - Verify that the cause of death was suicide.
   B. *Create an organizational culture that fosters positive connections between loss survivors and between loss survivors, leaders, and support personnel.*
      - Help create a school climate that fosters positive connections among students and between students and adults.
      - Report on activities coordinated by the local or state suicide prevention coalition.
      - Provide permission to grieve and a place to grieve.
      - Develop a safe climate within school districts.
      - Document actions taken.
      - Designate a crisis center area.
      - Legitimize and support the creation of a supportive social and cultural environment.
      - Document all information pertaining to the student's attempt, the school's follow-up, and the parents' response.
      - Establish a support center.
      - Make administrators and staff visible to students.
      - Keep an informal procedures log.
   C. *Develop a roster of decedents' family members.*
      - Identify full names of parents and guardians of schoolchildren.
      - Inform the school superintendent and administrators about siblings.

9. *Conduct gatekeeper training.* Support staff should receive "gatekeeper" training. Gatekeepers provide a link between at-risk individuals and mental health care providers or other resources.
   A. *Key personnel should receive gatekeeper training.*
      - Implement gatekeeper training on suicide prevention.
      - Verify that the cause of death was suicide.
      - Provide gatekeeper training for staff.
      - Train staff and students with Question, Prevent, Refer (emergency suicide gatekeeper training program) materials.
   B. *Train care providers to "connect" with grieving persons using the ATSM (Acute Traumatic Stress Management) model.*
      - Attempt to connect with the grieving person using the ATSM model.
      - Report on activities coordinated by the local or state suicide prevention coalition.
      - Provide permission to grieve and a place to grieve.

10. *Provide guidance for on-base death scenes.* Responders to a suspected suicide should not make judgments or punish witnesses for interfering with the body at the death scene.
   A. *Do not punish witnesses for interfering at the death scene.*
      - Do not lecture family on death scene procedures, particularly when they may have interfered (e.g., cut down a hanging body)
      - Verify that the cause of death was suicide.
   B. *Avoid making judgments at the death scene.*
      - Attempt to connect with the grieving person using the ATSM model.
      - Report on activities coordinated by the local or state suicide prevention coalition.
      - Provide permission to grieve and a place to grieve.

11. *Provide guidelines for leaders.* Leaders should reach out to loss survivors and demonstrate control while also consulting support staff to resolve internal concerns.
   A. *Leaders should develop a sense of mastery and control.*
      - Help develop a sense of mastery and control.
   B. *Leaders should discuss suicide details in a calm, clear, and concise manner.*
      - Remain calm and assure other students.
      - Discuss and establish a confidentiality protocol.
      - Communicate in a calm, informative, authoritative, and nurturing way.
      - Manage the situation and reduce "emotional contagion" (remain calm and reassuring).
      - Ensure that staff and teachers communicate with students as calmly as possible.
   C. *Leaders should reach out to interact with loss survivors about the suicide.*
      - Interact with students about the crisis.
      - Respect students' privacy. Share information with staff only as necessary.
      - "Be there" for the grieving person.
      - Comfort the grieving.
   D. *Leaders should consult with resource staff about concerns.*
      - Consult with school resource staff about concerns.

12. *Convey postvention messages strategically.* Messages delivered to various groups following a suicide should be delivered via several means (e.g., form letter, radio announcements, small-group notifications, personal messages), while the content of these messages should be concise and scripted in advance.
    A. *Communicate about suicides through personal modes.*
        - Inform students through personal communications.
    B. *Use multiple media (television, radio, Internet, social media) to convey messages.*
        - Use various forms of communication, including television and radio.
        - Remain calm and assure other students.
        - Discuss and establish a confidentiality protocol.
        - Identify several modes for both internal and external communication.
        - Communicate in a calm, informative, authoritative, and nurturing way.
    C. *Communicate about a suicide in small groups rather than a large-group setting.*
        - Do not release information during a large assembly or over the intercom.
        - Interact with students about the crisis.
        - Respect students' privacy. Share information with staff only as necessary.
        - Students should be informed in small-group settings in which questions can be answered, rumors dispelled, and concerns addressed.
        - "Be there" for the grieving person.
        - Comfort the grieving.
        - Inform students through discussion in small venues, not assemblies.
        - Schools or faith communities may consider organizing individual classes or small groups with adult leaders.
    D. *Notify organization members via letter.*
        - Inform parents and students about suicide and the school's response in a letter.
    E. *Do not conduct a mass assembly focusing on the decedent.*
        - Do not conduct mass assemblies focusing on decedent.
    F. *Communicate about suicides through letters prepared in advance.*
        - Supplement written communication to families and communities affected with other, oral communication and through the media (e.g., radio, television, community announcements).
        - Use prepared form letters.
    G. *Communicate quickly to key personnel first, if possible.*
        - Depending on the situation, communicate via a note to teachers and staff as quickly as feasible and in an open and clear manner.
    H. *Keep channels of communication open after a suicide.*
        - Depending on the situation, communicate via a note to teachers and staff as quickly as feasible and in an open and clear manner.
    I. *Keep conversations short.*
        - Keep conversations short.
    J. *Provide a script to support personnel (e.g., receptionists, secretaries).*
        - Provide secretaries with a script.
    K. *Provide fact sheets on grief.*
        - Provide facts about child survivors.
        - Provide facts about suicidal grief.
        - Provide facts about suicide loss survivors.

- Factual community briefs can help.

L. *Read announcements of the death to the entire organization.*
- Read school announcement of the death.

M. *Have a script for making death announcements.*
- Approve scripts for classroom announcements.
- Approve scripts for parent announcements.

13. *Allow loss survivors to convene.* Loss survivors should be encouraged to express grief in groups or alone, according to their individual needs.

A. *Care providers should personally visit the decedent's unit, class, or other organization to which he or she belonged.*
- Visit the deceased's classes.

B. *Allow individuals the opportunity to discuss the incident without input from leaders.*
- Provide opportunities for students to discuss concerns.
- Remain calm and assure other students.
- Discuss and establish a confidentiality protocol.

C. *Encourage multiple ways to express thoughts and feelings (e.g., writing, small-group discussions, one-on-one counseling).*
- Allow students to write letters or create a photo album of memories for the family.
- Allow students to channel their energy in constructive ways.
- Provide appropriate outlets for grieving, such as a display of prevention-related information or donations to the local crisis center.
- Provide an opportunity for small-group or individual discussion.

D. *Encourage individuals to talk with someone about their emotions.*
- Do not avoid questions.
- Inform parents and students about the suicide and the school's response in a letter.
- Share your feelings with someone you trust.
- Talk with someone about your emotions.
- Plan appropriate actions with the loss survivor to engage him or her in therapeutic interaction.

E. *Formally allow people to take time to grieve.*
- Take time to grieve.
- Tell loss survivors to "take things slowly" and take care of themselves and their families.

F. *Identify and provide tailored services to those who witnessed the suicide or discovered the body.*
- Identify those who have witnessed suicide or discovered the body.

G. *Make expressing one's thoughts voluntary.*
- Do not force participation.
- Depending on the situation, communicate via a note to teachers and staff as quickly as feasible and in an open and clear manner.
- Encourage emotional expression but do not insist.
- Do not pressure or force a conversation about the event.
- Do not force a discussion if students do not want to enter one.
- Do not insist on emotional expression.

- Do not require all students or staff to attend memorials.

H. *Provide psychological first aid.*
- Provide psychoeducation or psychological first-aid services for affected students and staff, as needed.
- Depending on the situation, communicate via a note to teachers and staff as quickly as feasible and in an open and clear manner.
- Triage injuries and provide emergency first aid to those who need it.

I. *Provide stress management during regularly scheduled assignments or duties.*
- Provide stress management time during class (allow students to express their feelings).

J. *Provide loss survivors with "alone time" or opportunities for silence.*
- Allow for alone time.
- Provide secretaries with a script.
- Allow periods of silence.

K. *Specifically reach out to those most affected.*
- Reach out to those most affected.
- Provide facts about child survivors.
- Recognize the unique challenges in grieving the loss of a loved one.
- Provide facts about suicidal grief.

14. *Encourage funeral or service participation.* Funeral service attendance and participation should be encouraged.

A. *Allow organization members time off to attend the funeral.*
- Encourage students, with parental permission, to attend the funeral.
- Visit the victim's classes.
- Encourage affected students, with parental permission, to attend the funeral.

B. *Offer transportation to the funeral.*
- Offer transportation to the place of worship or cultural center.

C. *Provide details about memorials, visiting hours, and funeral services in communicating about the suicide.*
- Provide information on community-based funeral services or memorials.
- Allow students to write letters or create a photo album of memories for the family.
- Communicate information about visiting hours and funeral services.
- Allow students to channel their energy in constructive ways.
- Relay information about funeral services.
- Provide appropriate outlets for grieving, such as a display of prevention-related information or donations to a local crisis center.

D. *Choose pallbearers and others involved in memorials or services with care.*
- Choose pallbearers with care.
- Inform parents and students about the suicide and the school's response in a letter.

15. *Ensure the necessary infrastructure.* Suicide response infrastructure—including funds, supplies, training, and policies—should be organized in advance of a suicide event, and the deployment of these resources should avoid adversely affecting normal routines following a suicide.
    A. *Have funds specifically allocated.*
        - Funding helps sustain programming.
        - Visit the victim's classes.
        - Set up interagency agreements to ensure that resources will be available.
    B. *Have policy guiding procedures.*
        - Set up a school board policy authorizing postvention activities.
    C. *Hold regular (e.g., annual) suicide prevention training.*
        - Incorporate suicide prevention into the curriculum.
        - Allow students to write letters or create a photo album of memories for the family.
    D. *Have supplies ready and organized.*
        - Keep supplies nearby and organized at all times.
        - Choose pallbearers with care.
        - Inform parents and students about the suicide and the school's response in a letter
        - Ensure that communication devices are compatible with emergency responder devices.
        - Ensure that schools have adequate communication gear.
    E. *Maintain a regular schedule after a suicide occurs.*
        - Return to normalcy as soon as possible.
        - Return to work with care.
        - Coping with a suicide might not require unique skills; rather, regular routines might be comforting.
        - Focus the immediate response on restoring equilibrium.
        - Help students return to normalcy.
        - Keep a regular schedule.
        - Reestablish routines.
        - Realize that life will return to normal.
        - Resume routines.
        - Keep the school open during normal hours.
        - Adjust schedules as necessary.
        - Do not cancel school for the funeral.
        - Return students to daily, predictable routines.
        - Return to the "business of learning" as soon as possible.
    F. *Provide care providers with professional development opportunities.*
        - Provide professional development opportunities for staff.
    G. *Conduct activities at all levels.*
        - Provide classroom interventions.

16. *Interact with family members appropriately.* Organizations should reach out to family members of both the decedent and loss survivors to make them aware of the suicide, the organizational response to the suicide, and available resources for support.
    A. *Reach out to the loss survivor's family.*
        - Notify parents via a letter.

- Notify parents or guardians.
- Notify siblings at other schools.
- Provide written notice to parents and teachers.
- Maintain contact with the loss survivor's parents regarding schoolwork.
- Contact parents to coordinate activities and assist in identifying resources.
- Inform parents through a group meeting.
- Provide written information to parents who need to be notified.
- Develop a school-family partnership.
- Arrange parent meetings.
- Inform parents or guardians about death and funeral.
- Follow up with parent or guardians.

B. *Reach out to the decedent's family.*
- Offer condolences to parents.
- Assure the family that what is happening is procedural, not personal.
- Contact the family.
- Arrange for school personnel to visit the family of the deceased.
- Follow up and support the family.
- Set up school board policy authorizing postvention activities.

C. *Describe the communication strategy to family members.*
- Communicate with family and community members about the memorial service.
- Provide the family with assistance with the memorial service.
- Offer assistance to the family and discuss the communication strategy.
- Keep parents and staff informed of upcoming activities.

D. *Provide resources to decedents' families.*
- Notify other students' parents online about the suicide.
- Provide materials for staff members and parents.
- Identify school district contacts for concerned family and parents.
- Recommend community-based mental health services to parents and guardians.

E. *Provide family members with information about how to help loss survivors grieve.*
- Provide educators and parents with information and behavioral strategies to help children in crisis.

F. *Have specific guidance and policies on notifying families when a decedent dies by suicide.*
- Create communication plans to notify families that a crisis has occurred.

G. *Hold meetings for spouses and children.*
- Provide classroom interventions.

H. *Notify family members of those deemed at risk.*
- Provide staff and parents with information about related behaviors.
- Warn parents about suicide risk.
- Always notify parents when there appears to be any risk of self-harm.

I. *Have specific guidance and policies on notifying families when a decedent dies by suicide.*
- Create communication plans to notify families that a crisis has occurred.

17. *Interact strategically with the media.* Effective and efficient communication and collaboration with the media can help to prevent additional suicides and increase community awareness of risk factors.
    A. *Handle discussions with media carefully.*
        - Work with a public relations coordinator on media communications.
        - Prearrange school liaisons to interact with parents, outside agencies, and the media.
    B. *Encourage media representatives to follow American Association of Suicidology guidelines.*
        - Encourage media representatives to follow American Association of Suicidology guidelines.
        - Focus media attention on actions individuals can take to prevent suicides by others.
        - Focus media attention on individual stories of how treatment was life-saving.
        - Focus media attention on myths about suicide.
        - Focus media attention on recent treatment advances.
        - Focus media attention on stories of people who overcame despair without attempting suicide.
        - Focus media attention on trends in suicide rates.
        - Focus media attention on the warning signs of suicide.
        - Assist the media in reporting responsibly and accurately.
    C. *Interact closely with the media after a suicide.*
        - Interact carefully with the media to avoid contagion.
    D. *Have a designated media spokesperson.*
        - Funnel all information through a public affairs officer.
        - Designate a media spokesperson.
        - Identify spokesperson as point of contact for concerned campus members and their families, as well as the media.
    E. *Have a strategy for responding to media requests.*
        - Develop a strategy for responding to media requests.

18. *Involve senior leaders.* Prepared leaders will help facilitate an effective response plan.
    A. *Advise leadership on postvention procedures.*
        - Advise the principal how to proceed.

19. *Conduct appropriate memorial services.* Memorials can provide an opportunity for loss survivors to support each other in their grief. The memorial should be designed to allow for healing and support for loss survivors, and possibly to try to prevent future suicides. Some guidelines directly conflict with one another in this category, however.
    A. *Ensure that memorials will not preclude discussions of grief and emotion.*
        - Do not schedule a memorial to preclude student discussions of grief and emotion.
    B. *Be prepared to handle youth needs before and after the memorial.*
        - Prepare for youth needs before and after memorial.
    C. *Avoid featuring tributes by friends or relatives.*
        - Avoid featuring tributes by friends or relatives.

D. *Discourage public personal expression (e.g., songs, poems).*
   - Discourage public personal expression (e.g., songs, poems).

E. *Identify acceptable types of memorials (e.g., permanent, physical memorials, activity-focused memorials, memorial services).*
   - Alternative strategies may include personal expressions given to the family and kept private or activity-focused memorials (e.g., day of community service, fundraising).
   - Conduct on-campus memorial services.
   - Consider a memorial activity.
   - Develop living memorials (e.g., tolerance programs).
   - Develop living memorials that will help students cope with their feelings.
   - Discourage on-campus physical memorials.
   - Do not allow a memorial to simply recount tales of the traumatic stressor.
   - Do not allow memorials to be a forum for anger and hate.
   - Do not assume "one size fits all" for memorials.
   - Do not conduct on-campus memorial services.
   - Do not create permanent memorials or dedications or hold a service on campus.
   - Do not dedicate memorials in public settings.
   - Do not dedicate yearbooks, songs, or sporting events to the suicide victim.
   - Do not establish a permanent memorial.
   - Do not focus the memorial on the uncontrollable aspects of the crisis.
   - Focus memorials on how to prevent future suicides.
   - If a memorial takes place, focus on positive messaging and emphasize solutions and support resources.
   - Limit memorials.
   - Memorials should be something to prevent other suicides.
   - A donation drive can help.
   - Avoid permanent markers and glamorization.
   - Consider appropriate types of public memorials.

F. *Encourage involvement in appropriate memorials.*
   - Encourage student involvement in living memorials that prevent other suicides.

G. *Hold a memorial after a suicide.*
   - A memorial or candle-lighting that follows safe messaging suggestions can be helpful.

20. *Do not use inappropriate words, terms, or images in communications.* It can be difficult to deliver accurate and effective messaging after a suicide because the reasons for the suicide are usually complex and not well understood. Messaging should not oversimplify the suicide or its causes and consequences, and it should not be judgmental or assign blame. It should be noted that some of these guidelines conflict with category 21, "Use appropriate words, terms, and images in communications."

    A. *Do not depict death as a positive end state.*
       - Do not say, "God wanted her/him more than you did."
       - Avoid featuring tributes by friends or relatives.
       - Do not say, "He's in a much better place now."
       - Do not say, "It was his/her time."

B. *Do not describe the suicidal act in communications with loss survivors.*
   - Acknowledge rumors and put them into context.
   - Discourage public personal expression (e.g., songs, poems).
   - Avoid reporting "how-to" description of suicide.
   - Do not describe the suicidal act.
   - Do not disclose extensive and disturbing detail about the means of death.
   - Limit information regarding a suicide.
   - Minimize exposure to upsetting images.

C. *Avoid sensationalizing, romanticizing, or glorifying the suicide decedent in communications with loss survivors.*
   - Avoid denial blaming, dramatizing, or glorifying the attempt.
   - Avoid glamorizing the suicide of a celebrity.
   - Avoid glorifying suicide or those who die by suicide.
   - Avoid glorifying suicide victims or sensationalizing them.
   - Do not glamorize or romanticize suicide.
   - Do not romanticize someone who has died by suicide.
   - Encourage parents and clergy to avoid glorifying the suicidal act.
   - The response should avoid glorifying victims and should minimize sensationalism.
   - Try to move students away from glamorizing or romanticizing the event.
   - Emphasize the accuracy and reality of tragic circumstances while avoiding unnecessarily gruesome details.
   - Avoid sensational coverage of suicide.
   - Do not glorify the suicide act or provide details.
   - Prevent imitation and modeling by avoiding glamorization of the current state of "peace" the decedent may have found.
   - To avoid glamorizing or sensationalizing the suicide, consider a comparison with past activities, use good taste, focus on the future, and respect the family's wishes.

D. *Do not rationalize the suicide.*
   - Avoid presenting suicide as a tool for accomplishing certain ends.

E. *Avoid blaming individuals or organizations for not preventing the suicide.*
   - Avoid absolution (e.g., "No one could have stopped it").

F. *Avoid blaming the decedent.*
   - Avoid blaming the decedent (e.g., "He should have been stronger").
   - Avoid being judgmental (e.g., "See what using gets you").
   - Remain nonjudgmental about the decedent.
   - Do not say, "Sometimes people make poor choices."
   - Do not say, "What a waste. How selfish of him."
   - Do not encourage or support blame.

G. *Avoid excessive, repetitive, or prominent reporting on suicide.*
   - Avoid excessive, repetitive, or prominent reporting on suicide.

H. *Avoid focusing only on the suicide decedent's positive characteristics.*
   - Avoid focusing only on the decedent's positive characteristics.
   - Separate positive qualities of the decedent's life from final act.

I. *Avoid oversimplifying the causes of suicide.*
   - Avoid oversimplifying the causes of suicide or presenting them as inexplicable or unavoidable.
   - Avoid simplistic explanations and clichés.
   - Avoid simplistic explanations of suicide.
   - Do not provide interpretations about motives or predictions about future events.

J. *Do not overstate the frequency of suicide in communications.*
   - Avoid overstating the frequency of suicide.
   - Do not present suicide as a common event but as a preventable tragedy.

21. *Use appropriate words, terms, and images in communications.* It can be difficult to deliver accurate and effective messaging after a suicide because the reasons for the suicide are usually complex and not well understood. Communication about the suicide can help loss survivors grieve, and obtain support, and it may even help prevent future suicides. It should be noted that some of these guidelines conflict with those in category 20, "Do not use inappropriate words, terms, or images in communications."

A. *Be sensitive when talking about the decedent.*
   - Talk about the decedent in a sensitive way.
   - Avoid featuring tributes by friends or relatives.

B. *Communicate stories about people who benefited from treatment.*
   - Include stories of people whose treatment was life-saving or who overcame despair.
   - Discourage public personal expressions (e.g., songs, poems).
   - Emphasize recent treatment advances for depression and mental illness.
   - Interview a mental health professional who is knowledgeable about suicide and treatment.

C. *Convey that the decedent is responsible for his or her actions.*
   - Convey that the victim is responsible for his or her actions.

D. *Provide loss survivors with a list of resources of people and organizations who can help.*
   - Find support.
   - Help students identify adults who can help.
   - Seek out supportive people.
   - Consider pointing out specific adults who are particularly resourceful and have a desire to help.
   - Encourage youth to identify adults they can rely on during times of crisis.
   - Let students know that help is available.
   - Provide referrals to community groups that can help.
   - Remind the student that school resource staff are available.
   - Include information about local crisis intervention services.
   - Share information on community resources.
   - Help identify resources.
   - Identify appropriate key figures in the community who can facilitate interactions.
   - Identify formal and informal community resources that address mental health needs.
   - Identify relevant community resources.
   - Identify resources that students may use.

- Assist in mobilizing a support system and share information about community services.
- Provide information about community resources.
- Provide information about resources within the school and community.
- Connect children with others in the community who are trustworthy and can help them cope.
- Learn about support groups.
- Provide resources to staff, students, parents, and the community.
- Seek out resources.

E. *Reach out to loss survivors and encourage them to utilize available resources.*
- Link at-risk students with community resources.
- Avoid absolution (e.g., "No one could have stopped it").
- Ask loss survivors about suicide responses directly and address concerns.
- Connect individuals with family, community, and peer support.
- Do not anticipate that students will seek out professional assistance.
- Encourage follow-through (i.e., see a family physician) as soon as possible.
- Encourage seeking specialized support.

F. *Provide truthful, factual information about the suicide.*
- Give straightforward information with a positive demeanor.
- Avoid blaming the victim (e.g., "He should have been stronger").
- Provide realistic and accurate information about the event in simple language.
- Avoid being judgmental (e.g., "See what using gets you").
- Provide timely, accurate, and appropriate information to the media.
- Remain nonjudgmental about the decedent.
- Be truthful and direct with students.
- Do not say, "Sometimes people make poor choices."
- Summarize the event and review predominant reactions; answer questions.
- Do not say, "What a waste. How selfish of him."
- Do not avoid discussions of the event.
- Do not encourage or support blame.
- Do not be deceptive or concealing.
- Elucidate with facts and control rumors.
- Circulate accurate information immediately to disrupt rumors and misinformation.
- Communicate information about the death.
- Communicate information about the decedent.
- Provide timely, accurate, and appropriate information to media.
- Provide updates with relevant facts as they become available.
- Verify the facts.
- Confirm the facts about the suicide.
- Communicate accurate and appropriate information.

G. *Relate decreasing trends in suicide rates over past decade.*
- Emphasize decreasing trends in national suicide rates over past decade.

H. *Stress alternatives to suicide in communications with loss survivors.*
- Stress alternatives to suicide.

I. *Take active steps to quash gossip related to the suicide.*
   - Avoid gossip about the causes.
   - Dispel rumors among the student body.

J. *Underscore the dangerous behavior of the decedent.*
   - Underscore the dangerous behavior of the decedent.

K. *Use appropriate language (i.e., "died by suicide" versus "committed" suicide, "successful" suicide, or "failed attempt").*
   - Avoid using "committed suicide" or "failed" or "successful" suicide attempt.
   - Use appropriate language (*not* "committed suicide," "successful suicide," or "failed attempt").
   - Use appropriate language (e.g., "died by suicide," "ended life").
   - Choose words carefully, respectfully, and lovingly.
   - Do not say, "He attempted suicide before he succeeded."
   - Do not say, "She committed suicide."
   - Say, "He died by suicide after a prior attempt."
   - Say, "She completed suicide" or "She died by suicide."

L. *Use consistent terminology across the organization.*
   - Use common terminology across the school district.

22. *Monitor community members and resources.* After a suicide, ongoing monitoring of supportive resources and potential high-risk groups and time periods might help providers efficiently deliver care to those in grief and prevent future suicides.

A. *Monitor, track, and intervene via social media outlets.*
   - Post suicide prevention resources on social media profiles.
   - Talk about the decedent in a sensitive way.
   - Avoid featuring tributes by friends or relatives.
   - Find social media profiles of the decedent and browse online conversations.

B. *Remain aware of holidays and anniversaries.*
   - Remain aware of holidays and anniversaries.
   - Include stories of people whose treatment was life-saving or who overcame despair.
   - Discourage public personal expression (e.g., songs, poems).
   - Emphasize recent treatment advances for depression and mental illness.
   - Prepare for secondary adversities and anniversaries.
   - Interview a mental health professional who is knowledgeable about suicide and treatment.
   - Review class lessons planned around anniversary dates.

C. *Remain aware of support groups.*
   - Remain aware of support groups.

D. *Sustain postvention support programs after the crisis has subsided.*
   - Continue intervention activities, groups, and follow-up.
   - Continue to make counseling available after the crisis has subsided.
   - Provide ongoing support as necessary.

23. *Protect loss survivors' privacy.* Suicide loss survivors should have privacy when dealing with their grief and should be protected from the media and its reports about the suicide.
    A. *Protect staff and loss survivors from the media.*
        - Protect staff members and students from the media.
        - Talk about deceased in sensitive way.
        - Avoid featuring tributes by friends or relatives.
    B. *Limit loss survivors' exposure to media reports.*
        - Limit media viewing.
        - Include stories of people whose treatment was life-saving or who overcame despair.
        - Discourage public personal expression (e.g., songs, poems).

24. *Create a response plan.* A thorough response plan should be thoughtfully developed and communicated to staff before a suicide. The plan should also be periodically reevaluated and adjusted if needed. This category includes guidance for developing various plan components.
    A. *Create an organizational postvention plan.*
        - The community should prepare a plan in advance.
        - Avoid featuring tributes by friends or relatives.
    B. *A postvention evaluation component should be part of a postvention plan.*
        - Evaluation tools can help determine impact.
        - Develop an evaluation component.
        - Evaluate responses.
    C. *Create an organization-specific postvention plan.*
        - Crisis planning helps organizations prepare for postvention.
        - Develop and follow a response plan.
        - Develop and implement a crisis plan or policy.
        - Develop a community response before a cluster onset.
        - Plan ahead.
        - Plan for recovery in the preparedness phase.
        - Prepare prevention, intervention, and postvention plans.
    D. *Conduct an assessment of the organizational response to a suicide (i.e., postvention evaluation).*
        - Assess the safety and integrity of facilities.
    E. *Allow some flexibility in implementing the crisis plan.*
        - Allow for flexibility in implementing the crisis plan.
        - Avoid absolution (e.g., "No one could have stopped it").
    F. *Conduct an assessment and determine the level of response needed.*
        - Assess the crisis and determine the level of crisis team involvement.
        - Assess the potential effect of the death.
        - Assess the potential impact on the school.
        - Assess the situation and choose the appropriate response.
        - Assess the emotional needs of staff, students, families, and responders.
        - Work in teams to assess the needs of loss survivors.
        - Estimate the level of response needed.

- Identify the scope of the crisis and plan for response at various time distances from the event.
- If implementing a plan, first contact and prepare key groups.
- Activate the crisis team. Verify the death and assess the impact on the school.
- Assemble assessment teams to monitor the needs of loss survivors.

G. *Convey messages to those who may be away from event (e.g., those who are deployed).*
- Identify those "away" from event or apart from those who share the loss.

H. *Determine beforehand what and how information will be shared.*
- Determine what and how information will be shared.
- Develop a communication plan for internal and external outreach.
- Establish clear lines of communication.
- Establish a notification process.
- Use planned communication channels.

I. *Have a timely response to a suicide.*
- Respond in a timely manner.
- Commence postvention immediately after the event.
- Initiate postvention within the first 24 hours following the death confirmation.
- Respond within seconds.
- Schedule a staff meeting as soon as possible.
- Take immediate action.

J. *Have an emergency safety plan during an acute crisis.*
- During a crisis, clear the area of other students immediately.
- Make regular school safety and security efforts part of mitigation and prevention practices.
- Promote security and a sense of safety.
- Ensure the physical safety of students and personnel, and arrange for medical care.
- Evacuate or lock down the school, as appropriate.
- Follow up with the security coordinator.
- Collaborate with the security coordinator regarding plans.

K. *Have procedures for handling donations.*
- Have procedures for handling donations.

L. *Implement a response plan for after a second traumatic death or a suicide cluster, versus a single suicide.*
- Implement a response plan for when a cluster occurs or when one or more traumatic deaths occur.
- The occurrence of either a suicide cluster or a death that might lead to a suicide cluster should trigger a response.
- Train faculty members, parents, and students to recognize warning signs and alert support services.

M. *Liaise with key personnel before beginning postvention activities.*
- Liaise with all relevant officials before beginning postvention efforts.

N. *Meet with key personnel immediately to review the postvention plan.*
- Meet with school staff as soon as possible to communicate next steps.
- Notify faculty and announce the staff meeting.

O. *Provide key personnel with advance notice.*
   ◦ Provide staff members with advance notice, if possible.

P. *Review postvention plans annually.*
   ◦ Develop an annual review of the postvention plan and revisions.
   ◦ Revisit the plan.

Q. *Have a coordinated notification plan.*
   ◦ Coordinate in-school notification.
   ◦ Create information-sharing processes.
   ◦ Inform faculty and staff.

R. *Have a prearranged system to guide how the local community will be informed of the death.*
   ◦ Announce the death to students through a prearranged system.
   ◦ Contact the superintendent.
   ◦ Notify other district schools.

S. *Notify affected individuals of the installation's crisis response plan.*
   ◦ Provide information about the school's crisis response plan.
   ◦ Provide information about the school's response.

25. *Establish a suicide response team.* A response team should be established prior to a suicide event. Team members should receive training, and each should have clearly defined roles and responsibilities. After the event, the team should debrief daily, and leaders should make an effort to appreciate those on the team.

A. *Appreciate those involved in crisis response.*
   ◦ Appreciate those involved in crisis response.
   ◦ Talk about the decedent in a sensitive way.
   ◦ Avoid featuring tributes by friends or relatives.

B. *Establish clear roles for members of the response team.*
   ◦ Define clear roles for the response team.
   ◦ Articulate clear roles for all involved in postvention.

C. *Have a daily debriefing after the death with the crisis response team.*
   ◦ Meet daily with the school-based crisis team.
   ◦ Schedule after-school debriefing sessions for staff.
   ◦ Plan to debrief postvention team members.
   ◦ Conduct daily debriefing.
   ◦ Debrief the postvention team.
   ◦ Debrief the response team and thank those who helped.
   ◦ Conduct daily debriefings for staff, responders, and others assisting in recovery.

D. *Identify members of a crisis intervention team and assign them specific postsuicide roles.*
   ◦ Identify members of a crisis intervention plan and assign them specific roles.
   ◦ Convene a crisis response team.
   ◦ Convene a crisis response team and provide support.
   ◦ Designate a student services staff member and hallway monitors.
   ◦ Designate school personnel to serve on the suicide prevention team.
   ◦ Develop a crisis team and a planning committee.
   ◦ Develop a suicide task force.
   ◦ Develop and train a crisis team.

- ◦ Develop and assign responsibilities and tasks.
- ◦ Involve all concerned sectors of the community, including a "coordinating" committee and a "host agency."

E. *Recruit and train a postvention team.*
- ◦ Mobilize a crisis response team.
- ◦ Mobilize the school-based crisis team.
- ◦ Organize crisis response team.
- ◦ Recruit and train members of the postvention team.
- ◦ Refresh training of district employees assigned to tragedy response.
- ◦ Delegate response activities.
- ◦ Plan to deploy key personnel during the postvention period.
- ◦ Back up team members with one to two potential replacements.

26. *Ensure that resources are available.* Ensure that mental health resources are available and accessible after a suicide.

A. *Mental health resources should be made readily available.*
- ◦ Mental health resources should be more readily available and easily accessible.
- ◦ Talk about the decedent in a sensitive way.
- ◦ Avoid featuring tributes by friends or relatives.

27. *Enforce rules and restrictions.* Specific to schools, students should not be permitted to leave the school building without official permission from parents and school administrators.

A. *Do not allow individuals to leave the institution without permission.*
- ◦ Allow students to leave school only with parental permission.
- ◦ Permit other students to leave school only with documented permission.

28. *Screen for high-risk individuals.* Formal screening procedures should be implemented after a suicide to identify individuals at increased suicide risk. Those identified as at risk should be referred to the appropriate resources.

A. *Be realistic about having leaders identify those needing mental health assistance.*
- ◦ Do not expect staff and faculty to independently identify individuals needing mental health assistance.
- ◦ Talk about the decedent in a sensitive way.
- ◦ Avoid featuring tributes by friends or relatives.

B. *Identify or screen high-risk individuals after the event and link them to services.*
- ◦ Evaluate psychological trauma risk.
- ◦ If suicidal behavior has been a "high-profile" event, debrief key students to provide fact-only information, diffuse anxiety, and emphasize positive reactions to stress.
- ◦ Identify students likely to be affected and refer them to services.
- ◦ Notify the parents of highly affected students.
- ◦ Implement gatekeeper training to help identify at-risk youth for interventions.
- ◦ Implement youth screening programs and classroom curriculum as part of prevention efforts.
- ◦ Implement a screening tool for the school district.

- Monitor and assist at-risk students.
- Monitor at-risk friends and students.
- Provide a referral system to identify at-risk youth.
- Have a detailed list of interventions for various levels of suicide risk: Level I, verbalization of suicide desire but no specific plans; Level II, plan for suicide and means to carry out plan; Level III, steps already taken to carrying out suicide.
- Develop a range of responsive services for at-risk students.
- Act immediately if concerned about suicide.
- Assess student risk of suicide by considering exposure.
- Assess suicidal student's level of risk.
- Identify and assess students who are at risk for suicide.
- Identify at-risk students in advance of anniversary dates or birthdays of deceased peers.
- Identify at-risk students and staff.
- Identify at-risk youth. Provide support and referrals when appropriate.
- Identify others at risk for suicide and conduct screening interviews.
- Identify students for follow-up by service staff.
- Be involved in identifying high-risk students.
- Individuals at high risk should be identified and receive at least one screening interview, plus follow-up counseling as needed.
- Screen loss survivors who need intensive follow-up care.
- Take any threat of self-harm seriously.
- Understand that the student is at high risk of another attempt.
- Notify parents and guardians of risk behaviors.
- Warn parents of suicide threats.
- Contact appropriate resources for students demonstrating self-violent behavior.
- Contact the police if safety is a concern.
- Follow up with the help of a mental health professional.
- If the risk is significant, stay with the student until help arrives.
- Inquire about mental illness.
- Refer students with concerning behavior to a counselor or the principal.
- Make support services available to at-risk students.

C. *Monitor individuals who may be less engaged in normal activities after a suicide.*
   - Record which students leave classroom.

D. *Take note of individuals with past problems (e.g., criminal justice, mental health, substance use).*
   - Identify problematic relationships with decedents.
   - Note students who may have alcohol or drug use issues.

E. *Screen for depression after a suicide.*
   - Offer depression screening for youth.

29. *Conduct suicide prevention training.* Suicide prevention education should be reiterated to external and internal communities after a suicide.

    A. *Educate members of the community about suicide prevention after a suicide.*
       - Explain the warning signs, protective and risk factors, and resources for help.
       - Increase school community awareness of suicide risk.

- Offer suicide prevention education.

B. *Tell loss survivors to watch others for signs of distress and emphasize the importance of letting someone know if they are concerned.*
- Encourage youth to watch each other for signs of distress and emphasize the importance of telling an adult if they suspect something.

C. *Inform staff about suicide warning signs.*
- Educate school personnel about warning signs and risk factors.
- Provide information to staff on warning signs.
- Review risk factors and warning signs with school faculty and support staff.
- Tell students that prevention is key and inform them about warning signs.

30. *Prepare counselors.* Those responsible for interacting with loss survivors should be prepared for varied responses to suicide, as well as varied responses to counseling.

A. *Be prepared for a range of emotional responses and surprises.*
- Expect a range of emotional responses from students.
- Expect to be surprised.
- Prepare for students' reactions.

B. *Identify long-term mental health needs.*
- Identify long-term mental health needs.

C. *Remind care providers that recovery may take time.*
- Do not attempt to simplify or expedite recovery.
- Take as much time as needed for recovery.

D. *Remind care providers that there may be unanswerable questions.*
- Acknowledge that there may be unanswerable questions.
- Understand difficult questions before answering them.

E. *Respect loss survivors' need to grieve and the intensity of emotions.*
- Respect the need to grieve and the intensity of emotions.
- Do not deny or dampen emotional responses.
- Do not underestimate the resurfacing of intense common grief reactions.
- Respect loss survivors' need to grieve.

31. *Use appropriate language with loss survivors.* This broad and vast category includes guidance on how to interact and what to say to loss survivors. Recommendations range from general (e.g., "There is no right way to feel after experiencing trauma") to specific (e.g., "Communicate the finality of death"). Advice is also provided on what to say (e.g., "Life is so unfair") and what not to say (e.g., inappropriate leveling: "I know how you feel"). Because some individuals may not feel comfortable or equipped to talk to loss survivors about their feelings and reactions to the suicide, resources for loss survivors (e.g., support groups, counselors) should be widely available and visible.

A. *Care providers should be clear about what can and cannot be done for loss survivors.*
- Be clear about what can and cannot be done for loss survivors.
- Do not try to accomplish all tasks in the school context.

B. *Acknowledge loss survivors' sense of loss and uncertainty.*
- It is best to acknowledge the sense of loss and uncertainty.
- Evaluation tools can help determine the impact.

C. *Avoid statements like "I know how you feel."*
   - Avoid inappropriate leveling (e.g., "I know how you feel").
D. *Avoid unrealistic expectations of loss survivors.*
   - Avoid unrealistic expectations (e.g., "You have to let him go now").
E. *Communicate that there is no "normal" reaction to suicide.*
   - There is no right way to feel after experiencing trauma.
   - Understand the uniqueness of suicide grief.
F. *Communicate the finality of death.*
   - Communicate the finality of death.
G. *Emphasize the finality of death in communications with loss survivors.*
   - Do not use clichés like "be strong" or "you're doing so well," which reinforce the individual's aloneness.
   - Emphasize the finality of death.
H. *Communicate the importance of social and family support.*
   - Contact with others can be useful.
   - Incorporate a peer support system.
   - Plan family time.
I. *Convey the message that feelings of anger, anxiety, and guilt are normal responses to a suicide.*
   - Assure loss survivors that feeling or expressing anger is a normal part of grieving.
   - Allow for the expression of anger and guilt.
   - Help students learn to manage anxiety that may result from a suicide.
   - Accept the intensity of the loss survivor's grief.
   - Anger is common.
   - Anxiety is normal.
   - Grief normalization: Reassure loss survivors that what they are feeling is normal.
   - Grieving individuals often go through various stages, including numbness, denial, dissociation, yearning and searching, disorganization, and reorganization.
   - It is normal to feel anxious.
   - Validate the student's reaction.
   - Normalize emotional reactions.
   - Help loss survivors deal with guilt.
   - Help loss survivors face anger.
   - Clarify that emotional responses are natural. Communicate that stress responses are normal reactions to abnormal situations.
   - Do not pathologize normal grief reactions.
   - Do not say, "All that anger will keep you from healing."
   - Do not say, "Don't feel guilty. You did all you could."
J. *Convey to loss survivors that suicide is often evidence of a mental illness.*
   - Inform the students that suicide is often evidence of mental illness.
K. *Discuss the event.*
   - Do not divert attention away from the event or dismiss its seriousness.
   - Recognize the loss.
L. *Emphasize the importance of seeking help when in need.*
   - Emphasize the complexity of suicide and the importance of help-seeking.

M. *Encourage loss survivors to attend to their physical health (e.g., get sleep, drink water, eat well, exercise, avoid increased use of alcohol, caffeine, or other substances).*
  - Avoid using or increasing the use of alcohol, caffeine, or other substances.
  - Drink plenty of water.
  - Drive safely.
  - Eat well and exercise.
  - Get plenty of rest.
  - Help maintain health and fitness.
  - Maintain good grooming.
  - Maintain proper diet and nutrition.
  - Reaffirm physical health and perceptions of security and safety.
  - Rest.

N. *Encourage loss survivors to develop coping strategies.*
  - Programs that focus on increasing problem solving, coping skills, and conflict resolution can increase resiliency and decrease suicide risk.
  - Build coping strategies.

O. *Encourage loss survivors to set goals.*
  - Encourage the goal of discovering constructive solutions to life's problems.
  - Focus on the needs and goals related to students.
  - Help loss survivors set realistic goals.
  - Convey long-term positive expectations.

P. *Encourage loss survivors in talking about the person who passed.*
  - Talk about the person who has passed.

Q. *Engage in positive, future-oriented activities.*
  - Get involved in positive activities.
  - Reorient children toward the future.
  - Emphasize signs of recovery and hope.
  - Reinforce positive coping strategies.
  - Channel student energy into projects that help the living, such as crisis hotline volunteering or service as peer helpers.

R. *Establish boundaries and rules.*
  - Establish boundaries and rules.

S. *Establish constraints for discussion outside therapy.*
  - Establish constraints for discussion outside therapy.

T. *Identify loss among marginalized or high-risk groups (e.g., children, estranged spouses, roommates).*
  - Help children and teens.
  - Identify traditionally marginalized loss survivors (e.g., common-law spouses, same-sex partners, estranged or divorced spouses, parents of adult victims, friends of young victims, roommates, support systems of those with mental illness, prisoners).

U. *Normalize help-seeking for emotional issues.*
  - Normalize the value of seeking professional help for emotional problems.
  - Introduce the topic of help-seeking.

V. *Do not be baited into an argument.*
  - Do not be baited into an argument.

W. *Do not overstate safety or provide false reassurance.*
- Do not overstate safety or provide false reassurance.
- Never give false assurances.

X. *Prevent others from discussing their own attempts.*
- Avoid first-person accounts from adolescents about their suicide attempts.

Y. *Provide therapeutic guidelines to care providers (e.g., do not minimize answers received, engage in reflective listening).*
- Be aware of body language, eye contact, and other communication techniques.
- Do not restate questions.
- Do not speculate.
- Do not be afraid to touch.
- Express sadness and feelings for affected loss survivors.
- Express warmth and nurturance.
- Listen.
- Use touch as encouragement and empathy.
- Say, "I'm here to support you whatever you are feeling."
- Express honest, genuine, and active interest and concern.
- Recognize the healing power of humor.
- Validate feelings, even if it is difficult.
- Do not minimize answers received.
- Listen to the answer.
- Paraphrase what you hear and repeat it back.
- Do not overestimate what the tragedy means.
- Establish rapport with the griever and extend offers of help.
- Help participants reflect upon any thoughts.

Z. *Provide loss survivors with an opportunity to express their thoughts and feelings.*
- Allow the bereaved to tell you how they feel, and try to normalize grief reactions.
- Allow students to discuss how they feel.
- Facilitate emotional expression.
- Help students talk about why a person dies by suicide.
- Permit discussion of emotions, and provide validation and support.

AA. *Provide time for loss survivors to write condolence letters.*
- Provide time and supplies for students to write condolence letters.

BB. *Remind loss survivors that painful feelings will decrease over time.*
- Remind loss survivors that painful feelings will decrease over time.

CC. *Respond to questions (avoid saying, "No comment").*
- "No comment" is not productive.

DD. *State that "life is so unfair."*
- Say, "Life is so unfair."

EE. *State that the suicide was "a tragedy."*
- Say, "What a tragedy."

FF. *Talk to loss survivors about how to deal with an "empty space."*
- Talk about how to deal with the empty chair.

GG. *Tell loss survivors to share their feelings about the loss with their families.*
- Share your feelings as a family.
- Share your reactions with your child.

HH. *Tell loss survivors they are not alone.*
  ◦ Help students understand they are not alone.
II. *Tell loss survivors to stay close with their families and friends.*
  ◦ Stay close to family and friends.

Excluded Recommendations: Focus on Suicide Attempters

- Support attempters with same kindness other persons in crisis receive.
- Offer support while trying to understand the event.
- Recommend counseling for the attempter and his or her family, and provide them with a list of community resources.
- Be available, demonstrate concern, maintain realistic expectations, provide perspective, and remain sensitive in response to the attempter and other students.
- Contact student services staff to meet with the student.
- Inform school liaisons about the attempt and have them inform the parents of the attempter, if necessary.
- Make every effort to facilitate the suicidal student's return to school.
- Maintain ongoing contact with the counseling agency as to treatment progress and goals (with signed release of consent).
- Ensure the physical health of the attempter.

Excluded Recommendations: Out of Scope

- Help children understand what might happen next and prepare for what's to come.
- Let friends give what they offer.
- Offer options for clothing disposal.
- Ask teachers and friends about your child.
- Refer to human services if neglect or abuse is suspected.
- Report suspected abuse.
- Adopt district-wide policies for suicide prevention.
- Appoint a host agency.
- Prevent other students from witnessing a traumatic event.
- Inform the building administrator.

Excluded Recommendations: Ill Defined

- Activate the student release system.
- Move the student from being a victim to an actor.
- Return to cognitive processing of the event.
- Treat all loss survivors the same way.
- Be specific.
- Be prepared for denial, dissociation, yearning or searching, disorganization, and reorganization.

- Counter denial.
- Envision a community with better or more resources.
- Envision a world in which the person could have benefited from care without stigma or prejudice.
- Provide break times.

Excluded Recommendations: Too Vague

- Encourage suicide prevention actions.
- Facilitate understanding of critical incident processing.
- Help provide closure when appropriate.
- Help loss survivors process their emotional reactions.
- Mitigate potential long-term psychological problems.
- Support.
- Offer to help.
- Reach out.
- Show compassion.
- Address young people directly by providing specific recommendations to unite the community.
- Funnel information to those caring for students.
- Keep students, families, and the media informed.
- Notify appropriate emergency responders and the school crisis team.
- Talk!
- Avoid clichés.
- Emphasize actions that communities can take to prevent suicides.
- Advocate for appropriate expressions of memorialization.
- Engage support staff and local crisis centers.
- Contact and prepare responder groups.
- Identify settings in which people are unable to express grief (e.g., prison, the military).
- Establish the infrastructure to provide assistance and support to students in need.
- Develop communications/media strategies.
- Provide guidance on structuring school activities.
- Notify the crisis team.
- Follow up.
- Follow up with the crisis team, staff, students, and parents.
- Police officers should receive better training.
- Provide helpful support.
- Consult with administrators, faculty members, and parents.
- Initiate a grief counseling plan.
- Long-term issues suggested by suicide should be addressed.
- Manage long-term reminders.
- Meet with school staff.
- Mobilize a pre-planned strategy to monitor and assist other students.
- Mobilize support and guidance.
- Notify district security office.

- Promote comprehensive suicide prevention in the community.
- Promote safety and respect in the school.
- Provide recommendations for community-based mental health services.
- Provide referrals.
- Reaffirm prevention efforts.
- Reflect with crisis response team and school personnel.
- Trust leadership.
- Concentrate on problem-solving.
- Conduct faculty planning sessions.
- Create a plan, assess, and follow up.
- Design mobilization criteria.
- Intervene as appropriate to prevent death.
- Prevent imitation and modeling.
- Prevent other crises from happening.
- Provide for aftermath interventions.
- Provide for post-crisis interventions.
- Provide interventions and respond to psychological needs.
- Remember to stay involved.
- Focus on loss survivor coping and efforts to prevent further suicides.
- Address long-term issues related to the suicide.
- Be careful with suicidal thoughts.
- Prevent and prepare for psychological trauma.

Excluded Recommendations: Other Reasons

- Young adults are remarkably resilient.
- Be flexible with body contact.
- Follow the deceased student's schedule to observe the reactions of students in his or her class.

Bibliography

Air Force Instruction 36-2910, *Line of Duty (Misconduct) Determination*, October 4, 2002, incorporating through change 2, April 5, 2010.

Air Force Instruction 36-3002, *Casualty Services*, February 22, 2010, certified current as of February 8, 2012.

Air Force Instruction 36-3009, *Airman and Family Readiness Centers*, May 7, 2013, incorporating change 1, December 4, 2013.

Air Force Mortuary Operations, "Families of the Fallen Support Branch," web page, undated. As of May 6, 2014:
http://www.mortuary.af.mil/library/familiesofthefallensupportbranch/index.asp

Andriessen, Karl, Annette Beautrais, Onja T. Grad, Elisabeth Brockmann, and Sue Simkin, "Current Understandings of Suicide Survivor Issues: Research, Practice, and Plans," *Crisis: The Journal of Crisis Intervention and Suicide Prevention*, Vol. 28, No. 4, 2007, pp. 211–213.

Aoun, Samar, "Deliberate Self-Harm in Rural Western Australia: Results of an Intervention Study," *Australian and New Zealand Journal of Mental Health Nursing*, Vol. 8, No. 2, June 1999, pp. 65–73.

Army Regulation 600-8-1, *Army Casualty Program*, April 30, 2007.

Army Regulation 600-8-4, *Line of Duty Policy, Procedures and Investigations*, September 4, 2008.

Army Regulation 600-20, *Army Command Policy*, March 18, 2008, rapid-action revision September 20, 2012.

Army Regulation 638-2, *Care and Disposition of Remains and Disposition of Personal Effects*, December 22, 2000.

Aseltine, Robert H., Jr., "An Evaluation of a School Based Suicide Prevention Program," *Adolescent and Family Health*, Vol. 3, No. 2, 2003, pp. 81–88.

Associated Press, "Army Will Investigate Recruiters' Suicides," *New York Times*, November 9, 2008, p. A32.

Baber, Kristine, and Gretchen Bean, "Frameworks: A Community-Based Approach to Preventing Youth Suicide," *Journal of Community Psychology*, Vol. 37, No. 6, August 2009, pp. 684–696.

Baird, Stephanie, and Sharon Rae Jenkins, "Vicarious Traumatization, Secondary Traumatic Stress, and Burnout in Sexual Assault and Domestic Violence Agency Staff," *Violence and Victims*, Vol. 18, No. 1, February 2003, pp. 71–86.

Baker, Thomas R., "Notifying Parents Following a College Student Suicide Attempt: A Review of Case Law and FERPA, and Recommendations for Practice," *NASPA Journal*, Vol. 42, No. 4, 2005, pp. 513–533.

Bean, Gretchen, and Kristine M. Baber, "Connect: An Effective Community-Based Youth Suicide Prevention Program," *Suicide and Life-Threatening Behavior*, Vol. 41, No. 1, February 2011, pp. 87–97.

Beck, Aaron T., Gregory K. Brown, Robert A. Steer, Katherine K. Dahlsgaard, and Jessica R. Grisham, "Suicide Ideation at Its Worst Point: A Predictor of Eventual Suicide in Psychiatric Outpatients," *Suicide and Life-Threatening Behavior*, Vol. 29, No. 1, Spring 1999, pp. 1–9.

Bidwell, R. E., J. J. Bidwell, and S. Y. Tsai, "Suicide Prevention: A Study of the Community Program in Kansas City," *Journal of the Kansas Medical Society*, Vol. 72, No. 4, April 1971, pp. 167–173 passim.

Birkhead, Guthrie S., Virginia G. Galvin, Patrick J. Meehan, Patrick W. O'Carroll, and James A. Mercy, "The Emergency Department in Surveillance of Attempted Suicide: Findings and Methodologic Considerations," *Public Health Reports*, Vol. 108, No. 3, May–June 1993, pp. 323–331.

Blue Ribbon Work Group on Suicide Prevention in the Veteran Population, *Report of the Blue Ribbon Work Group on Suicide Prevention in the Veteran Population*, Washington, D.C.: U.S. Department of Veterans Affairs, 2008.

Boelen, Paul A., Jos de Keijser, Marcel A. van den Hout, and Jan van den Bout, "Treatment of Complicated Grief: A Comparison Between Cognitive-Behavioral Therapy and Supportive Counseling," *Journal of Consulting and Clinical Psychology*, Vol. 75, No. 2, April 2007, pp. 277–284.

Bohanna, India, and Xiangdong Wang, "Media Guidelines for the Responsible Reporting of Suicide: A Review of Effectiveness," *Crisis*, Vol. 33, No. 4, 2012, pp. 190–198.

Bohus, Martin, Brigitte Haaf, Timothy Simms, Matthias F. Limberger, Christian Schmahl, Christine Unckel, Klaus Lieb, and Marsha M. Linehan, "Effectiveness of Inpatient Dialectical Behavioral Therapy for Borderline Personality Disorder: A Controlled Trial," *Behavioral Research and Therapy*, Vol. 42, No. 5, May 2004, pp. 487–499.

Bonnie, Richard J., Carolyn E. Fulco, and Catharyn T. Liverman, eds., *Reducing the Burden of Injury: Advancing Prevention and Treatment*, Washington, D.C.: National Academies Press, 1999.

Borowsky, Iris Wagman, Marjorie Ireland, and Michael D. Resnick, "Adolescent Suicide Attempts: Risks and Protectors," *Pediatrics*, Vol. 107, No. 3, March 2001, pp. 485–493.

Brent, David A., Mary Margaret Kerr, Charles Goldstein, James Bozigar, Mary Wartella, and Marjorie J. Allan, "An Outbreak of Suicide and Suicidal Behavior in a High School," *Journal of the American Academy of Child and Adolescent Psychiatry*, Vol. 28, No. 6, November 1989, pp. 918–924.

Brent, David A., Joshua A. Perper, Grace Moritz, Chris Allman, Joy Schweers, Claudia Roth, Lisa Balach, Rebecca Canobbio, and Laura Liotus, "Psychiatric Sequelae to the Loss of an Adolescent Peer to Suicide," *Journal of the American Academy of Child and Adolescent Psychiatry*, Vol. 32, No. 3, May 1993, pp. 509–517.

Brockhouse, Rebecca, Rachel M. Msetfi, Keren Cohen, and Stephen Joseph, "Vicarious Exposure to Trauma and Growth in Therapists: The Moderating Effects of Sense of Coherence, Organizational Support, and Empathy," *Journal of Traumatic Stress*, Vol. 24, No. 6, December 2011, pp. 735–742.

Brown, Ana C., Irwin N. Sandler, Jenn-Yun Tein, Xianchen Liu, and Rachel A. Haine, "Implications of Parental Suicide and Violent Death for Promotion of Resilience of Parentally-Bereaved Children," *Death Studies*, Vol. 31, No. 4, April 2007, pp. 301–335.

Brown, Gregory K., Thomas Ten Have, Gregg R. Henriques, Sharon X. Xie, Judd E. Hollander, and Aaron T. Beck, "Cognitive Therapy for the Prevention of Suicide Attempts: A Randomized Controlled Trial," *Journal of the American Medical Association*, Vol. 294, No. 5, August 3, 2005, pp. 563–570.

Bryan, Craig J., Luther E. Dhillon-Davis, and Kieran K. Dhillon-Davis, "Emotional Impact of a Video-Based Suicide Prevention Program on Suicidal Viewers and Suicide Survivors," *Suicide and Life-Threatening Behavior*, Vol. 39, No. 6, Dec, 2009, pp. 623–632.

Campbell, Frank R., Louis Cataldie, John McIntosh, and Kari Millet, "An Active Postvention Program," *Crisis*, Vol. 25, No. 1, 2004, pp. 30–32.

Carr, Russell B., "When a Soldier Commits Suicide in Iraq: Impact on Unit and Caregivers," *Psychiatry*, Vol. 74, No. 2, Summer 2011, pp. 95–106.

Cavanagh, J. T. O., A. J. Carson, M. Sharpe, and S. M. Lawrie, "Psychological Autopsy Studies of Suicide: A Systematic Review," *Psychological Medicine*, Vol. 33, No. 3, April 2003, pp. 395–405.

Center for Mental Health in Schools, University of California, Los Angeles, *Responding to Crisis at a School: A Resource Aid*, Los Angeles, Calif., 2008. As of May 6, 2014:
http://smhp.psych.ucla.edu/pdfdocs/crisis/crisis.pdf

Center for School Mental Health Assistance, University of Maryland, *Crisis Intervention: A Guide for School-Based Clinicians*, Baltimore, Md., 2002. As of May 6, 2014:
http://csmh.umaryland.edu/Resources/ResourcePackets/files/crisisintervention.pdf

Centers for Disease Control and Prevention, "CDC Recommendations for a Community Plan for the Prevention and Containment of Suicide Clusters," *Morbidity and Mortality Weekly*, Vol. 37, Suppl. 6, August 19, 1988, pp. 1–12. As of May 6, 2014:
http://wonder.cdc.gov/wonder/PrevGuid/p0000214/p0000214.asp

Centers for Disease Control and Prevention, National Institute of Mental Health, Office of the Surgeon General, Substance Abuse and Mental Health Services Administration, American Foundation for Suicide Prevention, American Association of Suicidology, and Annenberg Public Policy Center, *Reporting on Suicide: Recommendations for the Media*, New York: American Foundation for Suicide Prevention, 2002. As of May 6, 2014:
http://www.sprc.org/sites/sprc.org/files/library/sreporting.pdf

Centre for Evidence Based Medicine, "Oxford Centre for Evidence Based Medicine—Levels of Evidence (March 2009)," web page, last updated September 16, 2013. As of May 6, 2014:
http://www.cebm.net/?o=1025

Centre for Suicide Prevention, "School Memorials After Suicide: Helpful or Harmful?" *SEIC Alert*, No. 54, May 2004. As of May 6, 2014:
http://www.sprc.org/library_resources/items/school-memorials-after-suicide-helpful-or-harmful

———, "For Professionals: Considerations for School Settings," Calgary, Alb., 2005. As of May 6, 2014:
http://ww3.suicideinfo.ca/ForProfessionals/SchoolSettings/tabid/714/Default.aspx

Cerel, Julie, and Frank R. Campbell, "Suicide Survivors Seeking Mental Health Services: A Preliminary Examination of the Role of an Active Postvention Model," *Suicide and Life-Threatening Behavior*, Vol. 38, No. 1, February 2008, pp. 30–34.

Cerel, Julie, John R. Jordan, and Paul R. Duberstein, "The Impact of Suicide on the Family," *Crisis: The Journal of Crisis Intervention and Suicide Prevention*, Vol. 29, No. 1, 2008, pp. 38–44.

Cerel, Julie, Jason H. Padgett, Yeates Conwell, and Gerald A. Reed, "A Call for Research: The Need to Better Understand the Impact of Support Groups for Suicide Survivors," *Suicide and Life-Threatening Behavior*, Vol. 39, No. 3, 2009, pp. 269–281.

Chapple, A., and S. Ziebland, "Viewing the Body After Bereavement Due to a Traumatic Death: Qualitative Study in the UK," *British Medical Journal*, Vol. 340, No. 7754, May 8, 2010, pp. 1017–1028.

Cheung, Yee Tak Derek, Matthew J. Spittal, Michelle Kate Williamson, Sui Jay Tung, and Jane Pirkis, "Application of Scan Statistics to Detect Suicide Clusters in Australia," *PLoS One*, Vol. 8, No. 1, January 2013, p. e54168.

Cieslak, Roman, Kotaro Shoji, Aleksandra Luszczynska, Sandra Taylor, Anna Rogala, and Charles C. Benight, "Secondary Trauma Self-Efficacy: Concept and Its Measurement," *Psychological Assessment*, Vol. 25, No. 3, September 2013, pp. 917–928.

Collins, Sean, and Ann Long, "Too Tired to Care? The Psychological Effects of Working with Trauma," *Journal of Psychiatric Mental Health Nursing*, Vol. 10, No. 1, February 2003, pp. 17–27.

Colucci, Erminia, and Graham Martin, "Ethnocultural Aspects of Suicide in Young People: A Systematic Literature Review, Part 2: Risk Factors, Precipitating Agents, and Attitudes Toward Suicide," *Suicide and Life-Threatening Behavior*, Vol. 37, No. 2, April 2007, pp. 222–237.

Conner, Kenneth R., Annette L. Beautrais, David A. Brent, Yeates Conwell, Michael R. Phillips, and Barbara Schneider, "The Next Generation of Psychological Autopsy Studies, Part 1: Interview Content," *Suicide and Life-Threatening Behavior*, Vol. 41, No. 6, December 2011, pp. 594–613.

———, "The Next Generation of Psychological Autopsy Studies, Part 2: Interview Procedures," *Suicide and Life-Threatening Behavior*, Vol. 42, No. 1, February 2012, pp. 86–103.

Crosby, Alex E., LaVonne Ortega, and Cindi Melanson, *Self-Directed Violence Surveillance: Uniform Definitions and Recommended Data Elements*, Atlanta, Ga.: Centers for Disease Control and Prevention, February 2011.

Cutcliffe, John, and P. Bonny Ball, "Suicide Survivors and the Suicidology Academe: Reconciliation and Reciprocity," *Crisis: The Journal of Crisis Intervention and Suicide Prevention*, Vol. 30, No. 4, 2009, pp. 208–214.

Cvinar, Jacqueline G., "Do Suicide Survivors Suffer Social Stigma: A Review of the Literature," *Perspectives in Psychiatric Care*, Vol. 41, No. 1, January–March 2005, pp. 14–21.

Davidson, Kay W., and Zelda Foster, "Social Work with Dying and Bereaved Clients: Helping the Workers," *Social Work in Health Care*, Vol. 21, No. 4, 1995, pp. 1–16.

de Groot, Marieke H., Jos de Keijser, and Jan Neeleman, "Grief Shortly After Suicide and Natural Death: A Comparative Study Among Spouses and First-Degree Relatives," *Suicide and Life-Threatening Behavior*, Vol. 36, No. 4, August 2006, pp. 418–431.

de Groot, Marieke, Jos de Keijser, Jan Neeleman, Ad Kerkhof, Willem Nolen, and Huibert Burger, "Cognitive Behaviour Therapy to Prevent Complicated Grief Among Relatives and Spouses Bereaved by Suicide: Cluster Randomised Controlled Trial," *British Medical Journal*, Vol. 334, No. 7601, May 12, 2007, pp. 994–1000.

de Groot, Marieke, Jan Neeleman, Klaas van der Meer, and Huibert Burger, "The Effectiveness of Family-Based Cognitive-Behavior Grief Therapy to Prevent Complicated Grief in Relatives of Suicide Victims: The Mediating Role of Suicide Ideation," *Suicide and Life-Threatening Behavior*, Vol. 40, No. 5, October 2010, pp. 425–437.

De Leo, D., S. Burgis, J. M. Bertolote, A. J. Kerkhof, and U. Bille-Brahe, "Definitions of Suicidal Behavior: Lessons Learned from the WHO/EURO Multicentre Study," *Crisis*, Vol. 27, No. 1, 2006, pp. 4–15.

Dennis, M. L., M. Ives, and R. Funk, "GAIN-I Encyclopedia of Supplemental Documentation on Scales and Other Calculated Variables, Version 5.6," spreadsheet, Chestnut Health Systems, April 17, 2013.

Dennis, Michael, Janet C. Titus, Guy Diamond, Jean Donaldson, Susan H. Godley, Frank M. Tims, Charles Webb, Yifran Kaminer, Thomas Babor, M. C. Roebuck, Mark D. Godley, Nancy Hamilton, Howard Liddle, and Christy K. Scott, "The Cannabis Youth Treatment (CYT) Experiment: Rationale, Study Design and Analysis Plans," *Addiction*, Vol. 97, Suppl. 1, December 2002, pp. 16–34.

DoDI—*See* U.S. Department of Defense Instruction.

Dyregrov, Kari, "Assistance from Local Authorities Versus Survivors' Needs for Support After Suicide," *Death Studies*, Vol. 26, No. 8, 2002, pp. 647–668.

———, "What Do We Know About Needs for Help After Suicide in Different Parts of the World? A Phenomenological Perspective," *Crisis: The Journal of Crisis Intervention and Suicide Prevention*, Vol. 32, No. 6, 2011, pp. 310–318.

Eagle, Samantha, Aamy Creel, and Anne Alexandrov, "The Effect of Facilitated Peer Support Sessions on Burnout and Grief Management Among Health Care Providers in Pediatric Intensive Care Units: A Pilot Study," *Journal of Palliative Medicine*, Vol. 15, No. 11, November 2012, pp. 1178–1180.

Edwards-Stewart, Amanda, Julie T. Kinn, Jennifer D. June, and Nicole R. Fullerton, "Military and Civilian Media Coverage of Suicide," *Archives of Suicide Research*, Vol. 15, No. 4, 2011, pp. 304–312.

Evans, Robert, "Helping Students Cope with Suicide," fact sheet, Washington, D.C.: National Association of Independent Schools, June 25, 2004. As of May 6, 2014:
http://www.nais.org/Articles/Pages/Helping-Students-Cope-with-Suicide-145734.aspx

Etzersdorfer, Elmar, and Gernot Sonneck, "Preventing Suicide by Influencing Mass Media Reporting: The Viennese Experience 1980–1996," *Archives of Suicide Research*, Vol. 4, No. 1, 1998, pp. 64–74.

Etzersdorfer, Elmar, Gernot Sonneck, and Sibylle Nagel-Kuess, "Newspaper Reports and Suicide," *New England Journal of Medicine*, Vol. 327, No. 7, August 13, 1992, pp. 502–503.

Families for Depression Awareness, *Coping After a Suicide*, Waltham, Mass., 2008.

Farberow, Norman L., Han K. Kang, and Tim A. Bullman, "Combat Experience and Postservice Psychosocial Status as Predictors of Suicide in Vietnam Veterans," *Journal of Nervous and Mental Disease*, Vol. 178, No. 1, January 1990, pp. 32–37.

Feigelman, William, Bernard S. Gorman, Karyl Chastain Beal, and John R. Jordan, "Internet Support Groups for Suicide Survivors: A New Mode for Gaining Bereavement Assistance," *OMEGA: Journal of Death and Dying*, Vol. 57, No. 3, 2008, pp. 217–243.

Fikretoglu, Deniz, Stéphane Guay, David Pedlar, and Alain Brunet, "Twelve Month Use of Mental Health Services in a Nationally Representative, Active Military Sample," *Medical Care*, Vol. 46, No. 2, February 2008, pp. 217–223.

Foster, Tom, Kate Gillespie, Roy McClelland, and Chris Patterson, "Risk Factors for Suicide Independent of DSM-III-R Axis I Disorder: Case-Control Psychological Autopsy Study in Northern Ireland," *British Journal of Psychiatry*, Vol. 175, August 1999, pp. 175–179.

Fu, K. W., and P. S. F. Yip, "Changes in Reporting of Suicide News After the Promotion of the WHO Media Recommendations," *Suicide and Life-Threatening Behavior*, Vol. 38, No. 5, October 2008, pp. 631–636.

Gahm, Gregory A., Mark A. Reger, Julie T. Kinn, David D. Luxton, Nancy A. Skopp, and Nigel E. Bush, "Addressing the Surveillance Goal in the National Strategy for Suicide Prevention: The Department of Defense Suicide Event Report," *American Journal of Public Health*, Vol. 102, Suppl. 1, March 2012, pp. s24–s28.

Gibbons, Robert D., David C. Clark, and Jan Fawcett, "A Statistical Method for Evaluating Suicide Clusters and Implementing Cluster Surveillance," *American Journal of Epidemiology*, Vol. 132, No. 1, Suppl., July 1990, pp. s183–s191.

Goldsmith, S. K., T. C. Pellman, A. M. Kleinman, and W. E. Bunney, *Reducing Suicide: A National Imperative*, Washington, D.C.: National Academies Press, 2002.

Goode, Erica, "After Combat, Victims of an Inner War," *New York Times*, August 2, 2009, p. A1.

Goodkin, Karl, Nancy T. Blaney, Daniel J. Feaster, Teri Baldewicz, Jack E. Burkhalter, and Barbara Leeds, "A Randomized Controlled Clinical Trial of a Bereavement Support Group Intervention in Human Immunodeficiency Virus Type 1–Seropositive and –Seronegative Homosexual Men," *Archives of General Psychiatry*, Vol. 56, No. 1, January 1999, pp. 52–59.

Gordis, Leon, "Should Dead Cases Be Matched to Dead Controls?" *American Journal of Epidemiology*, Vol. 115, No. 1, January 1982, pp. 1–5.

Gould, Madelyn S., "Suicide and the Media," *Annals of the New York Academy of Science*, Vol. 932, April 2001, pp. 200–224.

Gould, Madelyn S., Frank A. Marrocco, Marjorie Kleinman, John Graham Thomas, Katherine Mostkoff, Jean Cote, and Mark Davies, "Evaluating Iatrogenic Risk of Youth Suicide Screening Programs: A Randomized Controlled Trial," *Journal of the American Medical Association*, Vol. 293, No. 13, April 6, 2005, pp. 1635–1643.

Gould, Madelyn S., Sylvan Wallenstein, and Lucy Davidson, "Suicide Clusters: A Critical Review," *Suicide and Life-Threatening Behavior*, Vol. 19, No. 1, Spring 1989, pp. 17–29.

Gould, Madelyn S., Sylvan Wallenstein, Marjorie H. Kleinman, Patrick O'Carroll, and James Mercy, "Suicide Clusters: An Examination of Age-Specific Effects," *American Journal of Public Health*, Vol. 80, No. 2, February 1990, pp. 211–212.

Grad, Onja T., Sheila Clark, Kari Dyregrov, and Karl Andriessen, "What Helps and What Hinders the Process of Surviving the Suicide of Somebody Close?" *Crisis: The Journal of Crisis Intervention and Suicide Prevention*, Vol. 25, No. 3, 2004, pp. 134–139.

Hacker, Karen, Jessica Collins, Leni Gross-Young, Stephanie Almeida, and Noreen Burke, "Coping with Youth Suicide and Overdose: One Community's Efforts to Investigate, Intervene, and Prevent Suicide Contagion," *Crisis: The Journal of Crisis Intervention and Suicide Prevention*, Vol. 29, No. 2, 2008, pp. 86–95.

Hall, Kristin M., "11 Suicides at Campbell Trigger Stand-Down," Associated Press, May 27, 2009. As of May 6, 2014:
http://www.armytimes.com/article/20090527/NEWS/905270341/11-suicides-Campbell-trigger-stand-down

Hallfors, Denise, Paul H. Brodish, Shereen Khatapoush, Victoria Sanchez, Hyunsan Cho, and Allan Steckler, "Feasibility of Screening Adolescents for Suicide Risk in 'Real-World' High School Settings," *American Journal of Public Health*, Vol. 96, No. 2, February 2006, pp. 282–287.

Hazell, Philip, and Terry Lewin, "An Evaluation of Postvention Following Adolescent Suicide," *Suicide and Life-Threatening Behavior*, Vol. 23, No. 2, Summer 1993, pp. 101–109.

Headquarters, U.S. Department of the Army, "Message: HQDA EXORD 103-09 ISO Army Suicide Prevention," memorandum, February 2009.

———, *Army Health Promotion, Risk Reduction, Suicide Prevention*, Washington, D.C., 2010.

———, *Army 2020: Generating Health and Discipline in the Force: Ahead of the Strategic Reset*, Washington, D.C., January 2012.

Henriksson, Markus M., Erkki T. Isometsä, Päivi S. Hietanen, Hillevi M. Aro, and Jouko K. Lonnqvist, "Mental Disorders in Cancer Suicides," *Journal of Affective Disorders*, Vol. 36, Nos. 1–2, December 1995, pp. 11–20.

Horowitz, Mardi J., Bryna Siegel, Are Holen, George A. Bonanno, Constance Milbrath, and Charles H. Stinson, "Diagnostic Criteria for Complicated Grief Disorder," *American Journal of Psychiatry*, Vol. 154, No. 7, July 1997, pp. 904–910.

Hourani, Laurel L., Giles Warrack, and Patricia A. Coben, "A Demographic Analysis of Suicide Among U.S. Navy Personnel," *Suicide and Life-Threatening Behavior*, Vol. 29, No. 4, Winter 1999, pp. 365–375.

Hsiung, Robert C., "A Suicide in an Online Mental Health Support Group: Reactions of the Group Members, Administrative Responses, and Recommendations," *CyberPsychology and Behavior*, Vol. 10, No. 4, 2007, pp. 495–500.

Husky, Mathilde M., Leslie McGuire, Laurie Flynn, Christine Chrostowski, and Mark Olfson, "Correlates of Help-Seeking Behavior Among At-Risk Adolescents," *Child Psychiatry and Human Development*, Vol. 40, No. 1, March 2009, pp. 15–24.

Jones, Lieutenant General Darrell D., statement to the Committee on Armed Services, U.S. House of Representatives, at the hearing "Status of Suicide Prevention Programs in the Air Force," Washington, D.C., September 9, 2011. As of May 6, 2014:
http://armedservices.house.gov/index.cfm/files/serve?File_id=aadda0e4-e7c0-4ad0-8571-665af22da557

Jobes, David A., Steven A. Wong, Amy K. Conrad, John F. Drozd, and Tracy Neal-Walden, "The Collaborative Assessment and Management of Suicidality Versus Treatment as Usual: A Retrospective Study with Suicidal Outpatients," *Suicide and Life-Threatening Behavior*, Vol. 35, No. 5, October 2005, pp. 483–497.

Jordan, John R., "Is Suicide Bereavement Different? A Reassessment of the Literature," *Suicide and Life-Threatening Behavior*, Vol. 31, No. 1, Spring 2001, pp. 91–102.

Jordan, John R., and John L. McIntosh, *Grief After Suicide: Understanding the Consequences and Caring for the Survivors*, New York: Routledge, 2011.

Keene, Elizabeth A., Nancy Hutton, Barbara Hall, and Cynda Rushton, "Bereavement Debriefing Sessions: An Intervention to Support Health Care Professionals in Managing Their Grief After the Death of a Patient," *Pediatric Nursing*, Vol. 36, No. 4, July–August, 2010, pp. 185–189.

Kerr, Mary Margaret, David A. Brent, Brian McKain, and Paula S. McCommons, *Postvention Standards Manual: A Guide for a School's Response in the Aftermath of Sudden Death*, 4th ed., Pittsburgh, Pa.: STAR Center, Division of Child Psychiatry, University of Pittsburgh Medical Center, 2010. As of May 6, 2014:
http://www.starcenter.pitt.edu/Files/PDF/Manuals/Postvention.pdf

Kersting, Anette, K. Kroker, J. Steinhard, K. Lüdorff, U. Wesselmann, P. Ohrmann, V. Arolt, and T. Suslow, "Complicated Grief After Traumatic Loss: A 14-Month Follow Up Study," *European Archives of Psychiatry and Clinical Neuroscience*, Vol. 257, No. 8, December 2007, pp. 437–443.

Klass, Dennis, "Developing a Cross-Cultural Model of Grief: The State of the Field," *OMEGA: The Journal of Death and Dying*, Vol. 39, No. 3, 1999, pp. 153–178.

Knox, Kerry L., David A. Litts, G. Wayne Talcott, Jill Catalano Feig, and Eric D. Caine, "Risk of Suicide and Related Adverse Outcomes After Exposure to a Suicide Prevention Programme in the US Air Force: Cohort Study," *British Medical Journal*, Vol. 327, No. 7428, December 13, 2003, pp. 1376–1381.

Knox, Kerry L., Barbara Stanley, Glenn W. Currier, Lisa Brenner, Marjan Ghahramanlou-Holloway, and Gregory Brown, "An Emergency Department–Based Brief Intervention for Veterans at Risk for Suicide (SAFE VET)," *American Journal of Public Health*, Vol. 102, Suppl. 1, March 2012, pp. s33–s37.

Kodaka, Manami, Vita Postuvan, Masatoshi Inagaki, and Mitsuhiko Yamada, "A Systematic Review of Scales That Measure Attitudes Toward Suicide," *International Journal of Social Psychiatry*, Vol. 57, No. 4, July 2011, pp. 338–361.

Krippendorff, Klaus, *Content Analysis: An Introduction to Its Methodology*, Thousand Oaks, Calif.: Sage Publications, 2004.

Kruesi, Markus J., Janet Grossman, James M. Pennington, Paul J. Woodward, David Duda, and Jay G. Hirsch, "Suicide and Violence Prevention: Parent Education in the Emergency Department," *Journal of the American Academy of Child and Adolescent Psychiatry*, Vol. 38, No. 3, March 1999, pp. 250–255.

Krysinska, Karolina, and Karl Andriessen, "On-Line Support and Resources for People Bereaved Through Suicide: What Is Available?" *Suicide and Life-Threatening Behavior*, Vol. 40, No. 6, December 2010, pp. 640–650.

Kuramoto, S. Janet, Bo Runeson, Elizabeth A. Stuart, Paul Lichtenstein, and Holly C. Wilcox, "Time to Hospitalization for Suicide Attempt by the Timing of Parental Suicide During Offspring Early Development," *JAMA Psychiatry*, Vol. 70, No. 2, February 2013, pp. 149–157.

Lamb, H. Richard, Linda E. Weinberger, and Walter J. DeCuir, Jr., "The Police and Mental Health," *Psychiatry Online*, Vol. 53, No. 10, October 2002.

Langford, Linda, David Litts, and Jane L. Pearson, "Using Science to Improve Communications About Suicide Among Military and Veteran Populations: Looking for a Few Good Messages," *American Journal of Public Health*, Vol. 103, No. 1, January 2013, pp. 31–38.

Lawyers.com, "Willful Misconduct and Your VA Benefits," web page, undated. As of May 6, 2014: http://military-law.lawyers.com/veterans-benefits/willful-misconduct-and-your-va-benefits.html

Leitner, Maria, Wally Barr, and Lindsay Hobby, *Effectiveness of Interventions to Prevent Suicide and Suicidal Behaviour: A Systematic Review*, Liverpool, Scotland: Scottish Government Social Research, January 2008.

Lerner, Mark D., and Raymond D. Shelton, "How Can Emergency Responders Help Grieving Individuals?" American Academy of Experts in Traumatic Stress, 2001.

Linehan, Marsha M., Katherine A. Comtois, Angela M. Murray, Martin Z. Brown, Robert J. Gallop, Heidi L. Heard, Kathryn E. Korslund, Darren A. Tutek, Sarah K. Reynolds, and Noam Lindenboim, "Two-Year Randomized Controlled Trial and Follow-Up of Dialectical Behavior Therapy vs Therapy by Experts for Suicidal Behaviors and Borderline Personality Disorder," *Archives of General Psychiatry*, Vol. 63, No. 7, July 2006, pp. 757–766.

Lohr, Kathleen N., "Rating the Strength of Scientific Evidence: Relevance for Quality Improvement Programs," *International Journal for Quality in Health Care*, Vol. 16, No. 1, February 2004, pp. 9–18.

Luoma, Jason B., Catherine E. Martin, and Jane L. Pearson, "Contact with Mental Health and Primary Care Providers Before Suicide: A Review of the Evidence," *American Journal of Psychiatry*, Vol. 159, No. 6, June 2002, pp. 909–916.

Maciejewski, Paul K., Baohui Zhang, Susan D. Block, and Holly G. Prigerson, "An Empirical Examination of the Stage Theory of Grief," *Journal of the American Medical Association*, Vol. 297, No. 7, February 21, 2007, pp. 716–723.

Maine Youth Suicide Prevention Program, "Media Guidelines for School Administrators Who May Interact with Reporters About Youth Suicide," fact sheet, 2007. As of May 6, 2014: http://www.maine.gov/suicide/professionals/program/mediaschool.htm

Mann, J. John, Alan Apter, Jose Bertolote, Annette Beautrais, Dianne Currier, Ann Haas, Ulrich Hegerl, Jouko Lonnqvist, Kevin Malone, Andrej Marusic, Lars Mehlum, George Patton, Michael Phillips, Wolfgang Rutz, Zoltan Rihmer, Armin Schmidtke, David Shaffer, Morton Silverman, Yoshitomo Takahashi, Airi Varnik, Danuta Wasserman, Paul Yip, and Herbert Hendin, "Suicide Prevention Strategies: A Systematic Review," *Journal of the American Medical Association*, Vol. 294, No. 16, October 26, 2005, pp. 2064–2074.

Mann, J. John, and Dianne Currier, "Evidence-Based Suicide Prevention Strategies: An Overview," in Maurizio Pompili and Roberto Tatarelli, eds., *Evidence-Based Practice in Suicidology: A Source Book*, Cambridge, Mass.: Hogrefe Publishing, 2011, pp. 67–87.

Marine Corps Order 1754.9, *Unit, Personnel and Family Readiness Program (UPFRP)*, February 9, 2012.

Marine Corps Order 3040.4, *Marine Corps Casualty Assistance Program*, March 1, 2011.

Maulik, Pallab K., William W. Eaton, and Catherine P. Bradshaw, "The Role of Social Network and Support in Mental Health Service Use: Findings from the Baltimore ECA Study," *Psychiatric Services*, Vol. 60, No. 9, September 2009, pp. 1222–1229.

McDaid, Catriona, Rebecca Trowman, Su Golder, Keith Hawton, and Amanda Sowden, "Interventions for People Bereaved Through Suicide: Systematic Review," *British Journal of Psychiatry*, Vol. 193, No. 6, December 2008, pp. 438–443.

McManus, Bonni L., Markus J. Kruesi, Arnim E. Dontes, Christian R. Defazio, John T. Piotrowski, and Paul J. Woodward, "Child and Adolescent Suicide Attempts: An Opportunity for Emergency Departments to Provide Injury Prevention Education," *American Journal of Emergency Medicine*, Vol. 15, No. 4, July 1997, pp. 357–360.

McMenamy, Jannette M., John R. Jordan, and Ann Mitchell, "What Do Suicide Survivors Tell Us They Need? Results of a Pilot Study," *Suicide and Life-Threatening Behavior*, Vol. 38, No. 4, August 2008, pp. 375–389.

Meadors, Patrick, and Angela Lamson, "Compassion Fatigue and Secondary Traumatization: Provider Self Care on Intensive Care Units for Children," *Journal of Pediatric Health Care*, Vol. 22, No. 1, January–February 2008, pp. 24–34.

Meehan, P. J., J. A. Lamb, L. E. Saltzman, and P. W. O'Carroll, "Attempted Suicide Among Young Adults: Progress Toward a Meaningful Estimate of Prevalence," *American Journal of Psychiatry*, Vol. 149, No. 1, January 1992, pp. 41–44.

Mental Health America of Wisconsin, *Garrett Lee Smith Youth Suicide Prevention Toolkit*, Milwaukee, Wisc., 2007.

———, *Community-Based Suicide Prevention Guidelines for Wisconsin*, Milwaukee, Wisc., 2010.

Metcalf, Peter, and Richard Huntington, *Celebrations of Death: The Anthropology of Mortuary Ritual*, Cambridge, UK: Cambridge University Press, 1991.

MHN Government Services, "Military and Family Life Counseling (MFLC) Program," web page, undated. As of May 6, 2014:
https://www.mhngs.com/app/programsandservices/mflc_program.content

Michel, Konrad, Kathrin Wyss, Conrad Frey, and Ladislav Valach, "An Exercise in Improving Suicide Reporting in Print Media," *Crisis: The Journal of Crisis Intervention and Suicide Prevention*, Vol. 21, No. 2, 2000, pp. 71–79.

Miller, Matthew, Catherine Barber, Melissa Young, Deborah Azrael, Kenneth Mukamal, and Elizabeth Lawler, "Veterans and Suicide: A Reexamination of the National Death Index–Linked National Health Interview Survey," *American Journal of Public Health*, Vol. 102, Suppl. 1, March 2012, pp. s154–s159.

Mishara, Brian L., Janie Houle, and Brigitte Lavoie, "Comparison of the Effects of Four Suicide Prevention Programs for Family and Friends of High-Risk Suicidal Men Who Do Not Seek Help Themselves," *Suicide and Life-Threatening Behavior*, Vol. 35, No. 3, June 2005, pp. 329–342.

Mitchell, A. M., T. Sakrida, B. Grabiak, and K. Barton, "An Investigation of Suicide Survivors' Perceptions of Bereavement Services," *Proceedings of the 38th Annual American Association of Suicidology Conference: Partnerships for Change: Advancing Suicide Prevention Services and Practices*, Broomfield, Colo.: American Association of Suicidology, 2005.

Montgomery County (Pa.) Emergency Medical Services, Inc., "After a Suicide: A Postvention Primer for Providers," *MCES Quest*, Vol. 5, No. 2, December 2006. As of May 6, 2014:
http://lifegard.tripod.com/After_a_Suicide.pdf

Morgan, H. G., E. M. Jones, and J. H. Owen, "Secondary Prevention of Non-Fatal Deliberate Self-Harm: The Green Card Study," *British Journal of Psychiatry*, Vol. 163, July 1993, pp. 111–112.

Motto, Jerome A., and Alan G. Bostrom, "A Randomized Controlled Trial of Postcrisis Suicide Prevention," *Psychiatric Services*, Vol. 52, No. 6, June 2001, pp. 828–833.

MyArmyBenefits, "Survivor Benefit Plan (SBP)," web page, last updated February 27, 2014. As of May 6, 2014:
http://myarmybenefits.us.army.mil/Home/Benefit_Library/Federal_Benefits_Page/Survivor_Benefit_Plan_(SBP).html?serv=147

National Action Alliance for Suicide Prevention, Clinical Care and Intervention Task Force, *Suicide Care in Systems Framework*, Washington, D.C., 2012.

National Association of School Psychologists, "Memorial Activities at School: A List of 'Dos' and 'Don'ts,'" fact sheet, 2002. As of May 6, 2014:
http://www.nasponline.org/resources/crisis_safety/memorialdo_donot.pdf

———, "Culturally Competent Crisis Response: Information for School Psychologists and Crisis Teams," fact sheet, 2004. As of May 6, 2014:
http://www.nasponline.org/resources/culturalcompetence/cc_crisis.pdf

National Suicide Prevention Lifeline, *Lifeline Online Suicide Prevention Manual*, Rockville, Md., 2010. As of May 6, 2014:
http://www.sprc.org/sites/sprc.org/files/library/LifelineOnlinePostventionManual.pdf

Navy Military Personnel Manual 1770, *Casualties and Survivor's Benefits*, August 8, 2006.

Navy Military Personnel Manual 1770-140, *Commanding Officer's Letter to Next of Kin*, August 22, 2002.

Neeleman, Jan, Simon Wessely, and Glyn Lewis, "Suicide Acceptability in African- and White Americans: The Role of Religion," *Journal of Nervous and Mental Disease*, Vol. 186, No. 1, January 1998, pp. 12–16.

Newson, Rachel S., Paul A. Boelen, Karin Hek, Albert Hofman, and Henning Tiemeier, "The Prevalence and Characteristics of Complicated Grief in Older Adults," *Journal of Affective Disorders*, Vol. 132, Nos. 1–2, July 2011, pp. 231–238.

Niederkrotenthaler, Thomas, and Gernot Sonneck, "Assessing the Impact of Media Guidelines for Reporting on Suicides in Austria: Interrupted Time Series Analysis," *Australian and New Zealand Journal of Psychiatry*, Vol. 41, No. 5, May 2007, pp. 419–428.

Niederkrotenthaler, T., M. Voracek, A. Herberth, B. Till, M. Strauss, E. Etzersdorfer, B. Eisenwort, and G. Sonneck, "Role of Media Reports in Completed and Prevented Suicide: Werther v. Papageno Effects," *British Journal of Psychiatry*, Vol. 197, No. 3, September 2010, pp. 234–243.

O'Connor, M., S. Nikoletti, L. J. Kristjanson, R. Loh, and B. Willcock, "Writing Therapy for the Bereaved: Evaluation of an Intervention," *Journal of Palliative Medicine*, Vol. 6, No. 2, April 2003, pp. 195–204.

O'Carroll, Patrick W., Alan L. Berman, Ronald W. Maris, Eve K. Moscicki, Bryan L. Tanney, and Morton M. Silverman, "Beyond the Tower of Babel: A Nomenclature for Suicidology," *Suicide and Life-Threatening Behavior*, Vol. 26, No. 3, Fall 1996, pp. 237–252.

O'Carroll, Patrick W., Alex Crosby, James A. Mercy, Roberta K. Lee, and Thomas R. Simon, "Interviewing Suicide 'Decedents': A Fourth Strategy for Risk Factor Assessment," *Suicide and Life-Threatening Behavior*, Vol. 32, No. 1, Suppl., 2001, pp. 3–6.

O'Carroll, Patrick W., and James A. Mercy, "Responding to Community-Identified Suicide Clusters: Statistical Verification of the Cluster Is Not the Primary Issue," *American Journal of Epidemiology*, Vol. 132, No. 1, Suppl., July 1990, pp. s196–s202.

O'Carroll, P. W., J. A. Mercy, and J. A. Steward, "CDC Recommendations for a Community Plan for the Prevention and Containment of Suicide Clusters," *Morbidity and Mortality Weekly Report*, Vol. 37, Suppl. 6, August 19, 1988, pp. 1–12.

Office of Safe and Drug-Free Schools, U.S. Department of Education, *Practical Information on Crisis Planning: A Guide for Schools and Communities*, Washington, D.C., 2007. As of May 6, 2014:
http://www2.ed.gov/admins/lead/safety/emergencyplan/crisisplanning.pdf

OPNAV Instruction 1754.1B, *Fleet and Family Support Center (FFSC) Program*, November 5, 2007.

Petcoff, Russell P., "Wingman Stand Down 2010 in May Focuses on Airmen Safety, Well-Being," Armed Forces News Service, April 30, 2010. As of May 6, 2014:
http://www.af.mil/News/ArticleDisplay/tabid/223/Article/116821/wingman-stand-down-2010-in-may-focuses-on-airmen-safety-well-being.aspx

Pfeffer, Cynthia R., Hong Jiang, Tatsuyui Kakuma, Judy Hwang, and Michele Metsch, "Group Intervention for Children Bereaved by the Suicide of a Relative," *Journal of the American Academy of Child and Adolescent Psychiatry*, Vol. 41, No. 5, May 2002, pp. 505–513.

Pierce, D. W., "The Predictive Validation of a Suicide Intent Scale: A Five Year Follow-Up," *British Journal of Psychiatry*, Vol. 139, No. 5, 1981, pp. 391–396.

Piper, William E., Mary McCallum, Anthony S. Joyce, John S. Rosie, and John S. Ogrodniczuk, "Patient Personality and Time-Limited Group Psychotherapy for Complicated Grief," *International Journal of Group Psychotherapy*, Vol. 51, No. 4, October 2001, pp. 525–552.

Piper, William E., John S. Ogrodniczuk, Anthony S. Joyce, Rene Weideman, and John S. Rosie, "Group Composition and Group Therapy for Complicated Grief," *Journal of Consulting Clinical Psycholology*, Vol. 75, No. 1, February 2007, pp. 116–125.

Pirkis, Jane, and R. Warwick Blood, "Suicide and the Media, Part I: Reportage in Nonfictional Media," *Crisis: The Journal of Crisis Intervention and Suicide Prevention*, Vol. 22, No. 4, 2001a, pp. 146–154.

———, "Suicide and the Media, Part II: Portrayal in Fictional Media," *Crisis: The Journal of Crisis Intervention and Suicide Prevention*, Vol. 22, No. 4, 2001b, pp. 155–162.

Pirkis, Jane, R. Warwick Blood, Annette Beautrais, Philip Burgess, and Jaelea Skehans, "Media Guidelines on the Reporting of Suicide," *Crisis: The Journal of Crisis Intervention and Suicide Prevention*, Vol. 27, No. 2, 2006, pp. 82–87.

Pirkis, Jane, Andrew Dare, R. Warwick Blood, Bree Rankin, Michelle Williamson, Philip Burgess, and Damien Jolley, "Changes in Media Reporting of Suicide in Australia Between 2000/01 and 2006/07," *Crisis: The Journal of Crisis Intervention and Suicide Prevention*, Vol. 30, No. 1, 2009, pp. 25–33.

Poland, Scott, and Donna Poland, "Dealing with Death at School," *Principal Leadership Magazine*, April 2004. As of May 6, 2014:
http://www.nasponline.org/resources/principals/Dealing%20with%20Death%20at%20School%20April%2004.pdf

Provini, C., J. R. Everett, and C. R. Pfeffer, "Adults Mourning Suicide: Self-Reported Concerns About Bereavement, Needs for Assistance, and Help-Seeking Behavior," *Death Studies*, Vol. 24, No. 1, 2000, pp. 1–19.

Public Law 103-160, National Defense Authorization Act for Fiscal Year 1994, November 30, 1993.

Public Law 108-136, National Defense Authorization Act for Fiscal Year 2004, November 24, 2003.

Public Law 108-375, National Defense Authorization Act for Fiscal Year 2005, October 28, 2004.

Public Law 109-163, National Defense Authorization Act for Fiscal Year 2005, January 6, 2006.

Public Law 109-364, National Defense Authorization Act for Fiscal Year 2007, October 17, 2006.

Public Law 110-417, National Defense Authorization Act for Fiscal Year 2009, October 14, 2008.

Radloff, Lenore Sawyer, "The Ces-D Scale," *Applied Psychological Measurement*, Vol. 1, No. 3, June 1977, pp. 385–401.

Rajagopal, Sundararajan, "Suicide Pacts and the Internet," *British Medical Journal*, Vol. 329, No. 7478, December 4, 2004, pp. 1298–1299.

Ramchand, Rajeev, Joie Acosta, Rachel M. Burns, Lisa H. Jaycox, and Christopher G. Pernin, *The War Within: Preventing Suicide in the U.S. Military*, Santa Monica, Calif.: RAND Corporation, MG- 953-OSD, 2011. As of May 6, 2014:
http://www.rand.org/pubs/monographs/MG953.html

Ramchand, Rajeev, Lynsay Ayer, Lilly Geyer, Aaron Kofner, C. Burnette, and Lila Rabinovich, *Gatekeepers in the Army and Marine Corps Suicide Prevention Program: Perspectives of NCOs and Chaplains*, Santa Monica, Calif.: RAND Corporation, forthcoming.

Ramchand, Rajeev, Nicole K. Eberhart, Christopher Guo, Eric Pederson, Terrance Dean Savitsky, Terri Tanielian, and Phoenix Voorhies, *Developing a Research Strategy for Suicide Prevention in the Department of Defense: Status of Current Research, Prioritizing Areas of Need, and Recommendations for Moving Forward*, Santa Monica, Calif.: RAND Corporation, RR-559-OSD, 2014. As of January 28, 2015: http://www.rand.org/pubs/research_reports/RR559.html

Recommendations for Reporting on Suicide, homepage, undated. As of May 6, 2014: http://reportingonsuicide.org

Reeves, Melissa A., Stephen E. Brock, Katherine C. Cowan, "Managing School Crises: More Than Just Response," *Principal Leadership Magazine*, May 2008. As of May 6, 2014: http://www.nasponline.org/resources/principals/School%20Crisis%20NASSP%20May%202008.pdf

Rosenberg, M. L., L. E. Davidson, J. C. Smith, A. L. Berman, H. Buzbee, G. Gantner, G. A. Gay, B. Moore-Lewis, D. H. Mills, and D. Murray, "Operational Criteria for the Determination of Suicide," *Journal of Forensic Sciences*, Vol. 33, No. 6, November 1988, pp. 1445–1456.

Rosenblatt, Paul C., "A Social Constructionist Perspective on Cultural Differences in Grief," in Margaret S. Stroebe, Robert O. Hansson, Wolfgang Stroebe, and Henk Schut, eds., *Handbook of Bereavement Research: Consequences, Coping, and Care*, Washington, D.C.: American Psychological Association, 2001, pp. 285–300.

Rutz, W., L. von Knorring, and J. Walinder, "Frequency of Suicide on Gotland After Systematic Postgraduate Education of General Practitioners," *Acta Psychiatric Scandinavica*, Vol. 80, No. 2, August 1989, pp. 151–154.

Ryan, Gery W., and H. Russell Bernard, "Techniques to Identify Themes," *Field Methods*, Vol. 15, No. 1, 2003, pp. 85–109.

Saarinen, Pirjo Irmeli, Heimo Viinamäki, Jukka Hintikka, Johannes Lehtonen, and Jouko Lönnqvist, "Psychological Symptoms of Close Relatives of Suicide Victims," *European Journal of Psychiatry*, Vol. 13, 1999, pp. 33–39.

Sabin-Farrell, Rachel, and Graham Turpin, "Vicarious Traumatization: Implications for the Mental Health of Health Workers," *Clinical Psychological Review*, Vol. 23, No. 3, May 2003, pp. 449–480.

Sandler, Irwin N., Yue Ma, Jenn-Yun Tein, Tim S. Ayers, Sharlene Wolchik, Cara Kennedy, and Roger Millsap, "Long-Term Effects of the Family Bereavement Program on Multiple Indicators of Grief in Parentally Bereaved Children and Adolescents," *Journal of Consulting and Clinical Psychology*, Vol. 78, No. 2, April 2010, pp. 131–143.

Schmidtke, Armin, and Sylvia Schaller, "The Role of Mass Media in Suicide Prevention," in Keith Hawton and Kees van Heeringen, eds., *The International Handbook of Suicide and Attempted Suicide*, Chichester, UK: John Wiley and Sons, 2000, pp. 675–697.

Scott, Michelle A., Holly C. Wilcox, Irvin Sam Schonfeld, Mark Davies, Roger C. Hicks, J. Blake Turner, and David Shaffer, "School-Based Screening to Identify At-Risk Students Not Already Known to School Professionals: The Columbia Suicide Screen," *American Journal of Public Health*, Vol. 99, No. 2, February 2009, pp. 334–339.

Shear, M. Katherine, "Complicated Grief Treatment: The Theory, Practice and Outcomes," *Bereavement Care*, Vol. 29, No. 3, December 2010, pp. 10–14.

Shear, M. Katherine, Ellen Frank, Patricia R. Houck, and Charles F. Reynolds, "Treatment of Complicated Grief: A Randomized Controlled Trial," *Journal of the American Medical Association*, Vol. 293, No. 21, June 1, 2005, pp. 2601–2608.

Shear, M. Katherine, Katie A. McLaughlin, Angela Ghesquiere, Michael J. Gruber, Nancy A. Sampson, and Ronald C. Kessler, "Complicated Grief Associated with Hurricane Katrina," *Depression and Anxiety*, Vol. 28, No. 8, August 2011, pp. 648–657.

Shear, M. Katherine, Naomi Simon, Melanie Wall, Sidney Zisook, Robert Neimeyer, Naihua Duan, Charles Reynolds, Barry Lebowitz, Sharon Sung, Angela Ghesquiere, Bonnie Gorscak, Paula Clayton, Masayo Ito, Satomi Nakajima, Takako Konishi, Nadeen Melhem, Kathleen Meert, Miriam Schiff, Mary-Frances O'Connor, Michael First, Jitender Sareen, James Bolton, Natalia Skritskaya, Anthony D. Mancini, and Aparna Keshaviah, "Complicated Grief and Related Bereavement Issues for DSM-5," *Depression and Anxiety*, Vol. 28, No. 2, February 2011, pp. 103–117.

Silverman, Morton M., Alan L. Berman, Nels D. Sanddal, Patrick W. O'Carroll, and Thomas E. Joiner, "Rebuilding the Tower of Babel: A Revised Nomenclature for the Study of Suicide and Suicidal Behaviors, Part 2: Suicide-Related Ideations, Communications, and Behaviors," *Suicide and Life-Threatening Behavior*, Vol. 37, No. 3, June 2007, pp. 264–277.

Sisask, Merike, and Airi Värnik, "Media Roles in Suicide Prevention: A Systematic Review," *International Journal of Environmental Research and Public Health*, Vol. 9, No. 1, January 2012, pp. 123–138.

Society for the Prevention of Teen Suicide, "For Parents," web page, undated. As of May 6, 2014:
http://www.sptsusa.org/parents/

SPRC—*See* Suicide Prevention Resource Center.

Stack, Steven, "Suicide in the Media: A Quantitative Review of Studies Based on Non-Fictional Stories," *Suicide and Life-Threatening Behavior*, Vol. 35, No. 2, April 2005, pp. 121–133.

Stanley, Barbara, and Gregory K. Brown, *The Safety Plan Treatment Manual to Reduce Suicide Risk: Veteran Version*, Washington, D.C.: U.S. Department of Veterans Affairs, 2008.

Strauss, Anselm C., and Juliet M. Corbin, *Basics of Qualitative Research: Techniques and Procedures for Developing Grounded Theory*, Thousand Oaks, Calif.: Sage Publications, 1998.

Substance Abuse and Mental Health Services Administration, "In the Wake of Trauma: Tips for College Students," Rockville, Md.: Substance Abuse and Mental Health Services Administration, 2010. As of May 6, 2014:
http://www.samhsa.gov/MentalHealth/AfterDisaster.pdf

Suich, Kaite, "Navy, Tragedy Assistance Program for Survivors Partner to Serve Navy Families," Navy News Service, May 26, 2011. As of May 6, 2014:
http://www.navy.mil/submit/display.asp?story_id=60641

Suicide Prevention Action Network USA and Suicide Prevention Resource Center, *Supporting Survivors of Suicide Loss: A Guide for Funeral Directors*, Washington, D.C., 2008. As of May 6, 2014:
http://www.sprc.org/sites/sprc.org/files/library/funeraldirectors.pdf

Suicide Prevention Resource Center, homepage, undated. As May 6, 2014:
http://www.sprc.org

———, *After a Suicide: Recommendations for Religious Services and Other Public Memorial Observances*, Newton, Mass.: Education Development Center, 2004. As of May 6, 2014:
http://www.sprc.org/sites/sprc.org/files/library/aftersuicide.pdf

———, "Best Practices Registry: Connect Suicide Prevention Training," web page, August 5, 2008. As of May 6, 2014:
http://www.sprc.org/bpr/section-III/connect-suicide-postvention-training

Sveen, Carl-Aksel, and Fredrik A. Walby, "Suicide Survivors' Mental Health and Grief Reactions: A Systematic Review of Controlled Studies," *Suicide and Life-Threatening Behavior*, Vol. 38, No. 1, February 2008, pp. 13–29.

Texas Suicide Prevention Community Network, *Coming Together to Care: A Suicide Prevention and Postvention Toolkit for Texas Communities*, Austin, Tex.: Mental Health America of Texas, July 2009. Updated version, as of May 6, 2014:
http://www.texassuicideprevention.org/wp-content/uploads/2013/06/TexasSuicidePrevention-2012Toolkit_8-31.pdf

Tragedy Assistance Program for Survivors, homepage, undated. As of May 6, 2014:
http://www.taps.org

TRICARE, "Eligibility," web page, last updated April 8, 2014. As of May 6, 2014:
http://www.tricare.mil/Welcome/Eligibility.aspx

Tuerk, Peter W., Matthew Yoder, Anouk Grubaugh, Hugh Myrick, Mark Hamner, and Ron Acierno, "Prolonged Exposure Therapy for Combat-Related Posttraumatic Stress Disorder: An Examination of Treatment Effectiveness for Veterans of the Wars in Afghanistan and Iraq," *Journal of Anxiety Disorders*, Vol. 25, No. 3, April 2011, pp. 397–403.

U.S. Army, "Survivor Benefit Plan," web page, last updated February 24, 2014. As of May 6, 2014:
http://myarmybenefits.us.army.mil/Home/Benefit_Library/Federal_Benefits_Page/Survivor_Benefit_Plan_(SBP).html

U.S. Department of the Army Pamphlet 600-24, *Suicide Prevention and Psychological Autopsy*, December 17, 2009, rapid-action revision September 7, 2010.

U.S. Army Family and Morale, Welfare and Recreation Command, homepage, undated. As of May 6, 2014:
http://www.army.mil/info/organization/unitsandcommands/commandstructure/fmwrc/

U.S. Department of Defense, *A Survivor's Guide to Benefits: Taking Care of Our Own*, Washington, D.C., current as of August 12, 2012. As of May 6, 2014:
http://www.militaryonesource.mil/12038/Project%20Documents/MilitaryHOMEFRONT/Casualty%20Assistance/Survivors%20Guide.pdf

U.S. Department of Defense Instruction 1300.18, Department of Defense (DoD) Personnel Casualty Matters, Policies, and Procedures, January 8, 2008, incorporating change 1, August 14, 2009.

U.S. Department of Defense Instruction 5154.30, *Armed Forces Institute of Pathology Operations*, March 18, 2003.

U.S. Department of Defense Instruction 5505.10, *Criminal Investigations of Noncombat Deaths*, August 15, 2013.

U.S. Department of Defense Task Force on the Prevention of Suicide by Members of the Armed Forces, *The Challenge and the Promise: Strengthening the Force, Preventing Suicide and Saving Lives*, Washington, D.C., August 2010.

U.S. Department of the Navy, Office of the Judge Advocate General, *Manual of the Judge Advocate General*, Washington, D.C., 2004.

U.S. Marine Corps Manpower and Reserve Affairs, "Casualty Assistant Calls Officer," web page, undated. As of May 6, 2014:
https://www.manpower.usmc.mil/portal/page/portal/M_RA_HOME/MF/C_PERSONNEL/Casualty/CACO

U.S. Preventive Services Task Force, homepage, undated. As of May 6, 2014:
http://www.uspreventiveservicestaskforce.org

Under Secretary of Defense for Personnel and Readiness, "Standardized DoD Suicide Data and Reporting," memorandum, June 18, 2006.

Van der Feltz-Cornelis, Christina M., Marco Sarchiapone, Vita Postuvan, Daniëlle Volker, Saska Roskar, Alenka Tancic Grum, Vladamir Carli, David McDaid, Rory O'Connor, Margaret Maxwell, Angela Ibelshäuser, Chantal Van Audenhove, Gert Scheerder, Merike Sisask, Ricardo Gusmão, and Ulrich Hegerl, "Best Practice Elements of Multilevel Suicide Prevention Strategies: A Review of Systematic Reviews," *Crisis: The Journal of Crisis Intervention and Suicide Prevention*, Vol. 32, No. 6, 2011, pp. 319–333.

van der Houwen, Karolijne, Henk Schut, Jan van den Bout, Margaret Stroebe, and Wolfgang Stroebe, "The Efficacy of a Brief Internet-Based Self-Help Intervention for the Bereaved," *Behaviour Research and Therapy*, Vol. 48, No. 5, May 2010, pp. 359–367.

Wagner, Birgit, Christine Knaevelsrud, and Andreas Maercker, "Internet-Based Cognitive-Behavioral Therapy for Complicated Grief: A Randomized Controlled Trial," *Death Studies*, Vol. 30, No. 5, June 2006, pp. 429–453.

Wasterlund, Michael, Sylvia Schaller, and Armin Schmidtke, "The Role of Mass-Media in Suicide Prevention," in Danuta Wasserman and Camilla Wasserman, eds., *Oxford Textbook of Suicidology and Suicide Prevention: A Global Perspective*, New York: Oxford University Press, 2009, pp. 515–523.

Weber, Robert Philip, *Basic Content Analysis*, 2nd ed., Newbury Park, Calif.: Sage Publications, 1990.

Werth, James L., Caroline Burke, and Rebekah J. Bardash, "Confidentiality in End-of-Life and After-Death Situations," *Ethics and Behavior,* Vol. 12, No. 3, 2002, pp. 205–222.

White House, Office of the Press Secretary, "Statement by the President on Change of Condolence Letter Policy," July 6, 2011. As of May 6, 2014:
http://www.whitehouse.gov/the-press-office/2011/07/06/statement-president-change-condolence-letter-policy.

Wilson, Anne, "Consumer Participation: Ensuring Suicide Postvention Research Counts for End Users," *International Journal of Nursing Practice,* Vol. 16, No. 1, February 2010, pp. 7–13.

Wittouck, Ciska, Sara Van Autreve, Eva De Jaegere, Gwendolyn Portzky, and Kees van Heeringen, "The Prevention and Treatment of Complicated Grief: A Meta-Analysis," *Clinical Psychology Review,* Vol. 31, No. 1, February 2011, pp. 69–78.

World Health Organization and International Association for Suicide Prevention, *Preventing Suicide: How to Start a Survivors' Group,* Geneva, Switzerland: World Health Organization Press, 2008. As of May 6, 2014:
http://www.who.int/mental_health/prevention/suicide/resource_survivors.pdf

Youth Suicide Prevention Program, "After a Suicide," fact sheet, 2003. As of May 6, 2014:
http://www.yspp.org/schools/crisis_response_after.htm